Problems in Otolaryngology

Problems in Practice Series

Problems in Practice Series

Series Editors : J.Fry K.G.D.Williams M.Lancaster-Smith

Problems
in
Otolaryngology

Padman Ratnesar
FRCS, FACS
Consultant Otolaryngologist
Farnborough Hospital, Kent

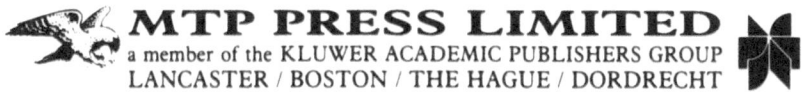

MTP PRESS LIMITED
a member of the KLUWER ACADEMIC PUBLISHERS GROUP
LANCASTER / BOSTON / THE HAGUE / DORDRECHT

Published by
MTP Press Limited
Falcon House
Lancaster, England

Copyright © 1984 MTP Press Limited
Softcover reprint of the hardcover 1st edition 1984

First published 1984

British Library Cataloguing in Publication Data

Ratnesar, P.
   Problems in otolaryngolgy. – (Problems in practice series)
   i. Otolaryngology
   I.Title II.Series
   616.2'2   RF46

   ISBN 978-94-011-6665-2   ISBN 978-94-011-6663-8 (eBook)
   DOI 10.1007/978-94-011-6663-8

Frome and London

Contents

5

Contents

Preface

The aim of this book is to give a short and practical account of the problems related to the ear, nose and throat. The presentation is orientated towards arriving at a diagnosis based on the presenting symptoms and signs and aid the management of the case. While it is specifically intended for those who have not had the opportunity of devoting much time to the subject, I hope that it may be of some service to the more experienced practitioner.

Padman Ratnesar
Farnborough, 1984

Series Foreword

This series of books is designed to help general practitioners. So are other books. What is unusual in this instance is their collective authorship; they are written by specialists working at district general hospitals. The writers derive their own experience from a range of cases less highly selected than those on which textbooks are traditionally based. They are also in a good position to pick out topics which they see creating difficulties for the practitioners of their district, whose personal capacities are familiar to them; and to concentrate on contexts where mistakes are most likely to occur. They are all well-accustomed to working in consultation.

All the authors write from hospital experience and from the viewpoint of their specialty. There are, therefore, matters important to family practice which should be sought not within this series, but elsewhere. Within the series much practical and useful advice is to be found with which the general practitioner can compare his existing performance and build in new ideas and improved techniques.

These books are attractively produced and I recommend them.

J. P. Horder CBE
Past President, The Royal College
of General Practitioners

1 Earache

Earache is frequent in practice. Probably more than 100 patients with earache see a general practitioner each year.

The causes may be in the external or middle ear or be referred from elsewhere.

External ear

Causes
There are common and rare causes of earache from the external ear. The common ones are acute otitis externa, furuncle, wax, foreign body and trauma. The rare causes are bullous myringitis, aural herpes, tumours and gout.

Otitis externa

Symptoms
This is a diffuse inflammatory condition (dermatitis) of the external meatus with swelling, redness, scaling and itching. Pain, deafness and discharge result. Extreme tenderness is felt on pulling the earlobe or touching the ear. Otitis externa affects young adults and those in early middle age.

Treatment is with:

(1) Systemic antibiotics – penicillin, ampicillin or erythromycin.

11

Treatment (2) Local insertion of magnesium sulphate paste with 1 ml syringe.

(3) Local insertion of corticosteroid drops.

Many of the severe cases will respond to antibiotics and these should be used before painful local procedures are carried out.

Furuncles

If these are very painful then systemic antibiotics – pencillin or erythromycin – are best.

Wax

Pain from ear wax is most often the result of attempts to dislodge or remove it by patient or doctor. Impacted wax should be softened by olive oil or sodium bicarbonate ear drops and then gently washed out.

Foreign bodies

If the body is impacted the patient should be referred to a consultant.

If it is not impacted gentle syringing may be tried.

Middle ear

Causes Common causes of earache from the middle ear are acute otitis media and serous (secretory) otitis media. Rarely it is caused by acute mastoiditis.

Acute otitis media

A general practitioner will see 50 children each year with acute otitis media or serous otitis. The conditions predominantly affect children.

Symptoms Clinical presentations are earache, fever and malaise, deafness and discharge.

Treatment relates to the individual severity of the case. A

12

Treatment   well child with a red drum needs analgesics only. A sick child
             with a red drum should be given antibiotics such as ampicillin,
             amoxycillin or co-trimoxazole. In all cases the patients should
             be followed up until drum and hearing return to normal.

Table 1.1   Possible causes of referred earache

Possible cause	Nerve supply
5th cranial nerve temporomandibular dysfunction impacted wisdom teeth parotid swellings	External auditory canal Pars flaccida
9th cranial nerve tonsillitis cancer of posterior one third of tongue	Typanic membrane External auditory canal
10th cranial nerve cancer of pyriform fossa	External auditory canal
Cervical 2nd and 3rd nerve roots spondylosis	Pinna External auditory canal

Serous (secretory) otitis

'Glue' presents with dull ache and deafness. It is seen
commonly in children but also affects adults. The drum is
retracted, yellow or bluish with prominent vessels. (See Figure
2.3). In children it is associated with dysfunction of the
Eustachian tube following upper respiratory infections. In
adults unilateral 'glue ear' may rarely be associated with a
nasopharyngeal tumour. Many cases resolve naturally without
operative interference. Those that do not resolve may require
Treatment   myringotomy, grommets and/or adenoidectomy.

Acute mastoiditis

Acute mastoiditis is now very rare in general practice.
It is not as 'acute' as its title suggests. It presents 10–14 days
after an acute otitis media with persisting ear discharge and ill
health and fever. Deafness and tenderness of mastoid X-rays
show clouding of the mastoid antrum.

Initial treatment is with intensive systemic antibiotics. If
there is no response, exploration and drainage of the mastoid is
necessary.

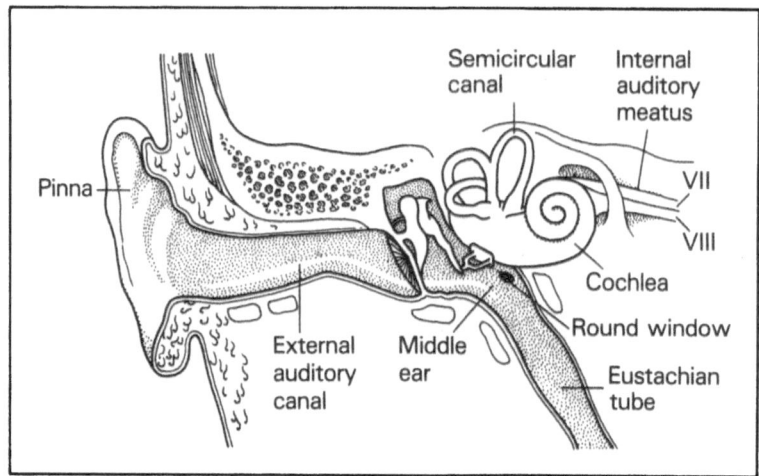

Figure 1.1   Diagram of outer/middle/inner ear which explains referred pain

Referred pain

Referred pain in the ear results from irritation of the 5th, 9th or 10th cranial nerves or the 2nd and/or 3rd cervical nerve roots (Table 1.1 and Figure 1.1). The nerve supply to two unrelated areas by the same nerve is referred to as dual innervation. Thus we find that the 5th, 9th and 10th cranial nerves and the 2nd and 3rd cervical nerves innervate structures of the pinna, external auditory canal and tympanic membrane. Thus a symptom related to structure other than the ear manifests as earache. This is illustrated in Figure 1.1.

2 Deafness

Types of hearing loss – Conductive deafness – Sensorineural deafness

Partial deafness or total loss of hearing may accompany earach, otorrhoea, vertigo or tinnitus.

History   The patient's history is important in order to determine the effects of the hearing loss in the patient. The history should include the age of onset (important for the development of language), the rate of onset, the severity of loss, whether the loss is unilateral or bilateral, and any associated factors especially congenital disorders or metabolic disorders, such as diabetes.

Types of hearing loss

Conductive deafness

Sensorineural loss

There are two main types of hearing loss, firstly conductive which is due to a disorder affecting the outer or middle ear, and secondly sensorineural loss which is a defect in the cochlea, nerve pathway or even the central nervous system. Sometimes the patient may have a *mixed type* of deafness which is a sensorineural loss with an added conductive element.

It is essential to understand the type of deafness to be able to correct the disorder, especially when rehabilitation with a hearing aid is considered.

15

Conductive deafness

Conductive deafness is due to a disorder affecting the outer and middle ear. It may be congenital or acquired due to a mechanical defect. The causes of conductive deafness could be grouped under anatomical sites, namely the external auditory canal, the tympanic membrane, and the middle ear and Eustachian tube.

External meatus

Wax or foreign body
Wax or a foreign body is the commonest cause in the external auditory canal. This is easily removed manually or after instilling olive oil by syringing. If this fails the patient should be referred to a hospital.

Inflammatory process
The inflammatory process of the external meatus should be either circumscribed – furunculosis – or diffuse when it is referred to as otitis externa. The commonest organism is a staphyloccal infection, though otitis externa is commonly seen in patients with diabetes. Sometimes the inflammatory process is due to a fungus infection.

Meatal stenosis
Meatal stenosis and, more obviously, congenital atresia of the external auditory canal are rare but still seen. The patient should be referred to an otologist for necessary investigation and management.

Trauma
Trauma to the external auditory canal following a road traffic accident, boxing or other sport can cause deafness due not only to obstruction by blood clots but also by lacerated tissue in the canal. Trauma is treated conservatively with systemic antibiotics and referred to the otologist for necessary investigations like X-rays and audiograms.

New growths
New growths of the external meatus may be benign or malignant. The conductive deafness is often due to discharge from the ear or even wax which is prevented from moving out of the canal. Bony exostosis of the external auditory canal can also behave like benign new growths to produce a conductive hearing loss. Although bony extosis is seen commonly, benign new growths, like papilloma and fibroma are rare and malignant growths like epithelioma, ceruminoma and sarcoma are more rare.

Benign
Malignant

Once these new growths are identified, the patient should be referred to an otologist for the necessary treatment.

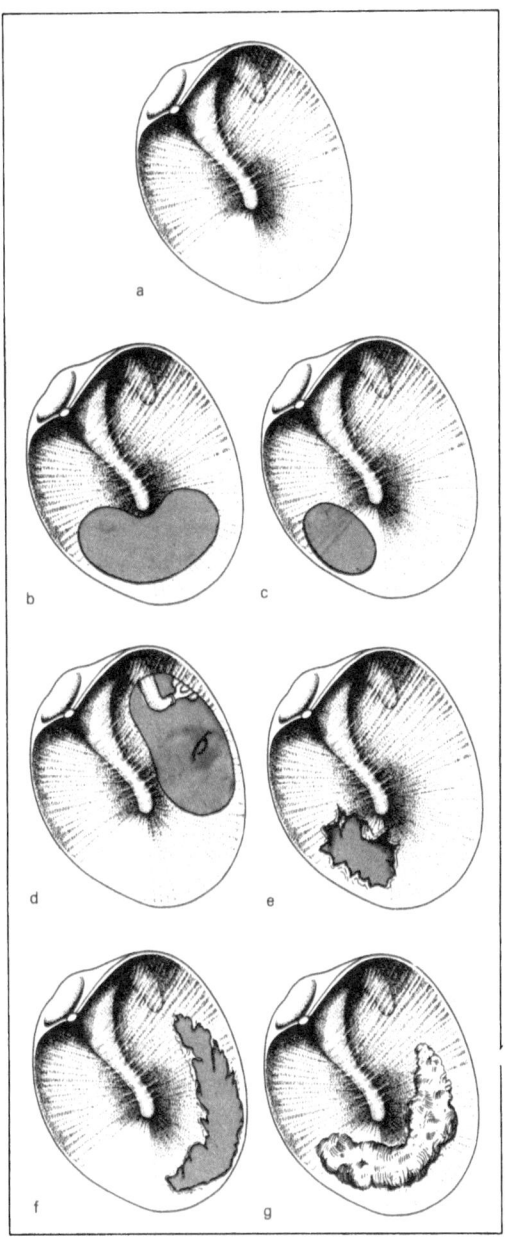

Different types of perforation. (a) Normal typanic membrane of the left ear; (b) central perforation; (c) anterio-inferior perforation; (d) posterior marginal perforation; (e) anterio-inferior traumatic perforation; (f) posterior traumatic perforation showing the ragged edges; (g) tympanosclerosis

Figure 2.1

Tympanic membrane

Perforations of the tympanic membrane interferes with the
Perforation · conduction of sound to the inner ear resulting in a conductive
hearing loss.

In identifying the perforation, the nature of site, size and
edges of the perforation gives an indication to its cause. The
history is also important especially in relation to trauma and
History · also whether the deafness was of sudden onset or gradual and
whether accompanied by bleeding or discharge. The degree of
deafness will not only be dependent on the size of the perforation, but also the accompanying features like discharge and
defects within the middle ear, i.e. ossicular damage.

The different types of perforation one often meets in a
practice are illustrated in Figure 2.1. The central and anterioin-
Different · ferior perforations are generally considered safe and are due to
types · tubotympanic disease, while the posterior and posteriomar-
ginal are unsafe and often due to atticoantral disease.

Tympanosclerosis of the tympanic membrane which is calci-
fication following hyaline change of the tympanic membrane,
Tympano- · does give rise to conductive hearing loss. The tympanic mem-
sclerosis · brane shows evidence of chalky patches which may coalesce.

Middle ear

Defects in the middle ear which result in a conductive hearing
loss could be the result of:
Defects
(1)   Acute inflammatory process and its sequelae.

(2)   Disruption of the ossicular chain due to trauma.

(3)   Congenital and hereditary disorders.

The commonest cause of acute inflammation of the middle
ear is the common cold and any upper respiratory infection can
Acute · spread to the middle ear cleft. The inflammatory process
inflammation · resulting in obstruction of the Eustachian tube results in the
collection of exudate in the middle ear called serous otitis
media, commonly seen in children but also in adults.

The earliest sign on the tympanic membrane is the loss of
light reflex. Depending on the amount of fluid in the middle
Loss of light · ear, on clinical examination it may present with a hair line or
reflex · air bubbles or injected drumhead or even bulging as shown in
Figure 2.2.

18

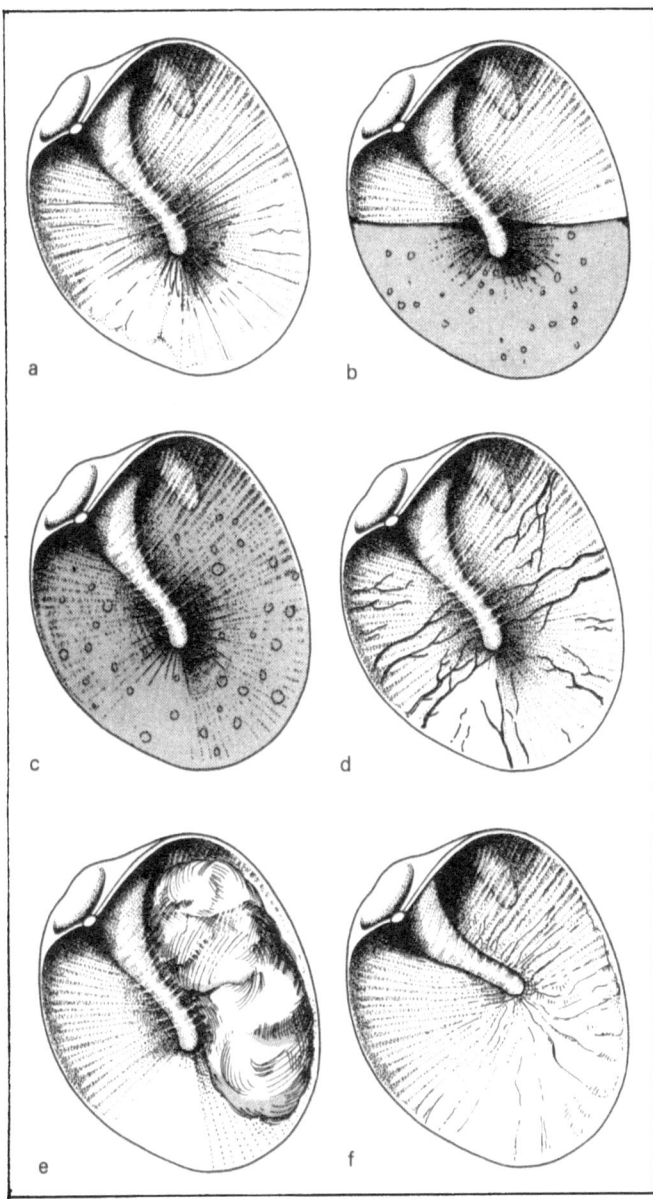

Appearance of the tympanic membrane. (a) early serous otitis also called acute Eustachian salpingitis; (b) fluid level in the ear in serous otitis showing the hair line; (c) fluid in the ear with air bubbles; (d) prominent blood vessels referred to as injected drumhead; (e) bulging tympanic membrane often seen in the posterior segment; (f) retracted tympanic membrane in glue ear with the short process of malleus rotated laterally

Figure 2.2

19

'Glue' ear

As the viscosity of the fluid increases it forms the 'glue' ear and the tympanic membrane may appear retracted and golden yellow in colour or blue due to previous haemorrhage.

Management is both medical and/or surgical.

Head injury

Head injury giving rise to a transverse or longtitudinal fracture through the temporal bone could give rise to a conductive deafness due to disruption of the ossicular chain or even a perceptive deafness due to damage of the cochlea.

Incus

The commonest ossicle to be fractured is the incus which may be dislocated from the stapes due to a fracture of the long process or even lie free in the middle ear.

Following the treatment of the head injury the conductive deafness can only be corrected by surgical procedure. Hence the patient should be referred to an otologist.

Congenital disorders of the middle ear are rare but the disorder of otosclerosis is much more common and thought to be hereditary.

Otosclerosis

Otosclerosis is a localized bone disease which commonly starts on the promontory in front of the oval window and spreads slowly to involve the margins of the oval window and ultimately fixes the footplate of the stapes, and involves the cochlea, though sometimes the cochlea alone may be affected. (Figure 2.3)

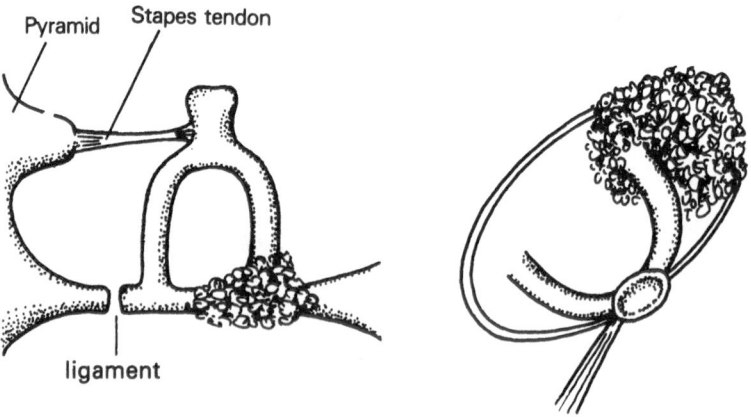

The otosclerotic changes usually start around the anterior crura and then spread to the rest of the footplate of the stapes

Figure 2.3

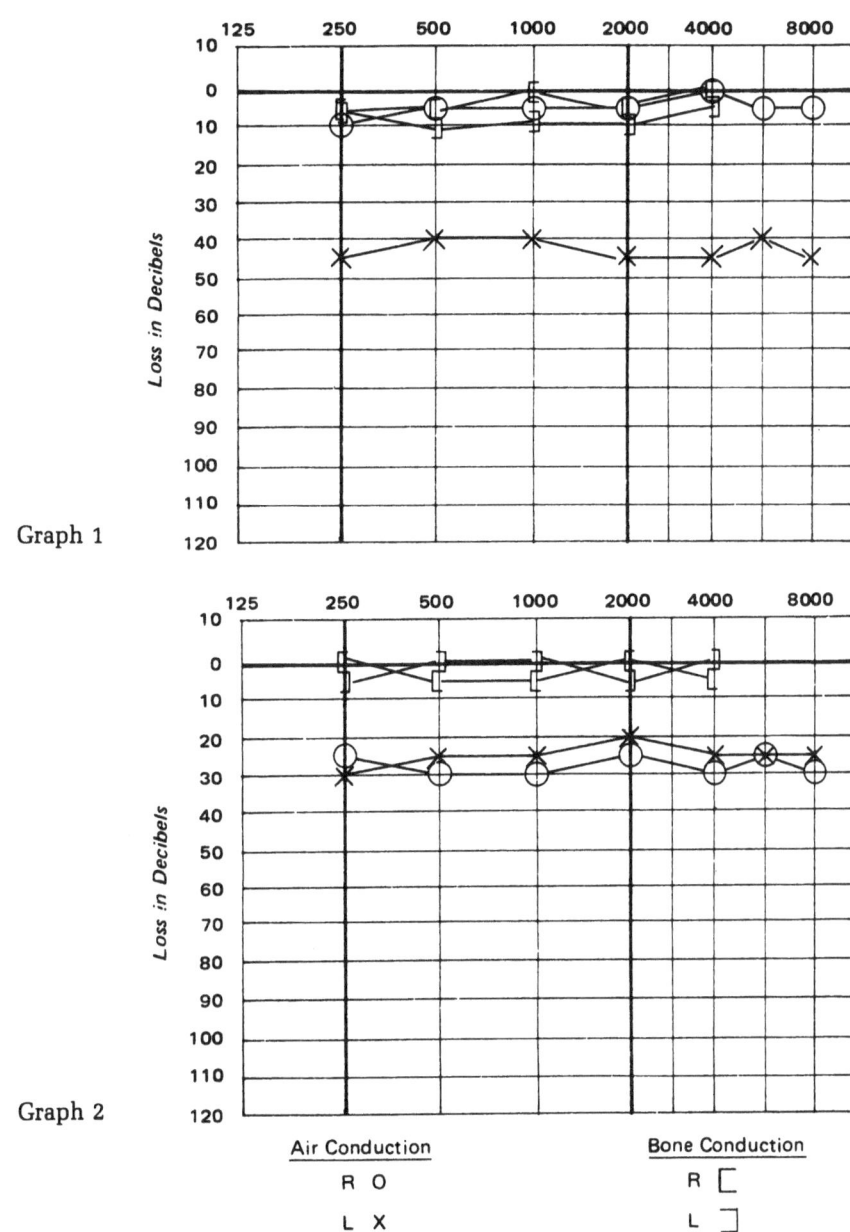

Graph 1

Graph 2

Air Conduction		Bone Conduction
R O		R ⊏
L X		L ⊐

Audiograms taken of patients with conductive deafness. (Graph 1) Unilaterial conductive hearing loss; (Graph 2) Bilateral conductive hearing loss; (Graph 3) Bilateral conductive hearing loss with unilateral perceptive element; (Graph 4) Mixed deafness showing high frequency loss

Figure 2.4

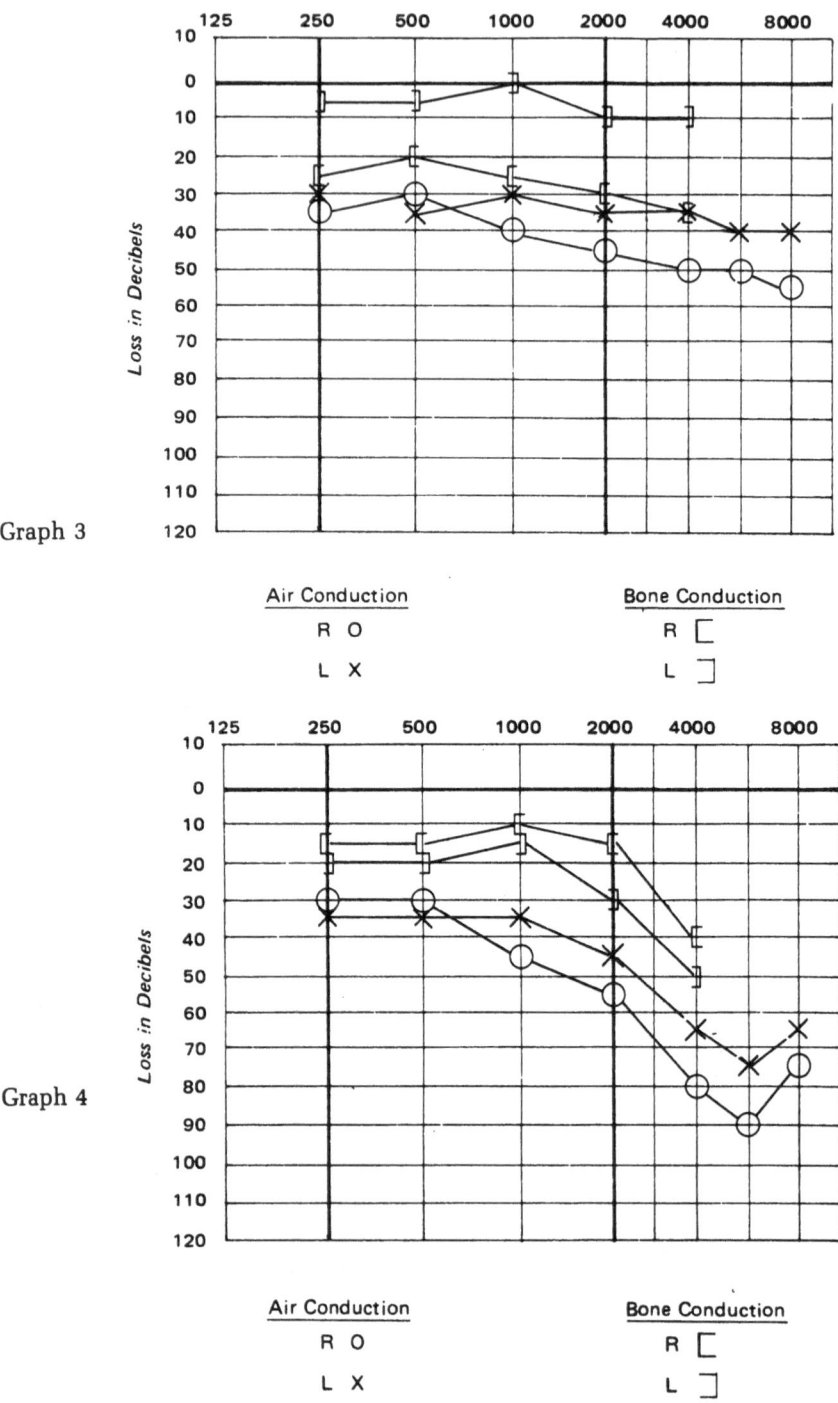

Graph 3

Air Conduction

R O

L X

Bone Conduction

R ⊏

L ⊐

Graph 4

Air Conduction

R O

L X

Bone Conduction

R ⊏

L ⊐

Otosclerosis accounts for about 50% of all cases of bilateral conductive hearing loss. Deafness is noticed in the third decade more commonly in females than males and often deafness is worse with each childbirth.

Since otosclerosis is a slowly progressive deafness the patient may not notice the disability till very late, although the individual may be aware of the deafness when the hearing falls to about 30–35 dB (see Figure 2.4).

Slow progression

Though the type of deafness is of a conductive nature, it is important to identify a perceptive element, nerve deafness, because it plays an important role in deciding if there is a place for surgery.

Surgery

Figure 2.4 shows that the patients with graphs 1 and 2 are suitable for surgery but the patient with graph 3 is suitable for surgery only in one ear and the patient with graph 4 is not suitable for surgery at all. Nevertheless, at present with good hearing aids available in the National Health Service and the private sector, a hearing aid would be suitable for types 2, 3 and 4.

Hearing aids

Although conductive deafness due to acute inflammatory process has been discussed in this chapter, to avoid repetition conductive deafness due to chronic inflammatory process will be discussed in Chapter 3 along with otorrhoea.

The following table helps to distinguish an inflammatory process of the external auditory canal from that of the middle ear cleft.

Table 2.1

Furunculosis	Acute mastoid disease
Onset and course rapid.	Onset gradual – about 2-3 weeks after middle ear infection.
Pain – intense, made worse by pressure and movement of temporo-mandibular joint	Only pain when pressure over body of mastoid.
Auricle may be swollen and projects outwards.	Auricle normal, but projects downwards and outwards from head.
External meatus obstructed by localized swelling, tender on probing.	External meatus swollen due to general thickening.

Table 2.1   (Continued)

The *discharge* is slight.	*Discharge* is profuse.
Drum seen to in intact.	*Drum* perforated.
Hearing usually normal.	*Hearing* usually marked deafness.

Effects of middle ear inflammation

The author's own work on the inter-relationship between different inflammatory processes and their sequelae is summarized in Tables 2.2 and 2.3. The conductive deafness due to either acute otitis media or serous otitis media may resolve with conservative treatment, whereas conductive deafness as a sequelae of chronic otitis media more often than not will need surgical intervention. Though the deafness may not be corrected, the principle is to give the patient a clean, dry ear.

Sensorineural deafness

Any disorder affecting the inner ear or the pathway in the nerve supply to the ear or even affecting the nucleus of the eighth nerve will cause a perceptive hearing loss often referred to as nerve deafness or sensorineural deafness. Figure 2.5 shows a typical audiogram from sensorineural deafness.

There are two main groups to sensorineural deafness, the congenital deafness and acquired sensorineural deafness.

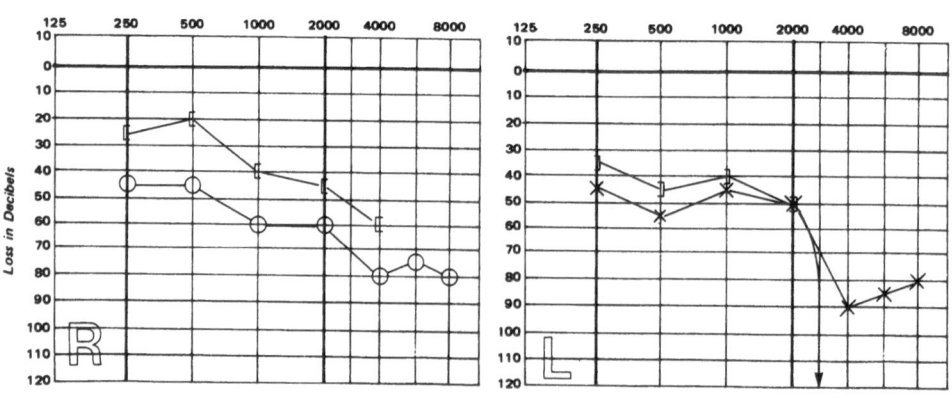

Audiogram from a patient with sensorineural deafness

Figure 2.5

Table 2.2 Inter-relation between different inflammatory processes and their sequelea

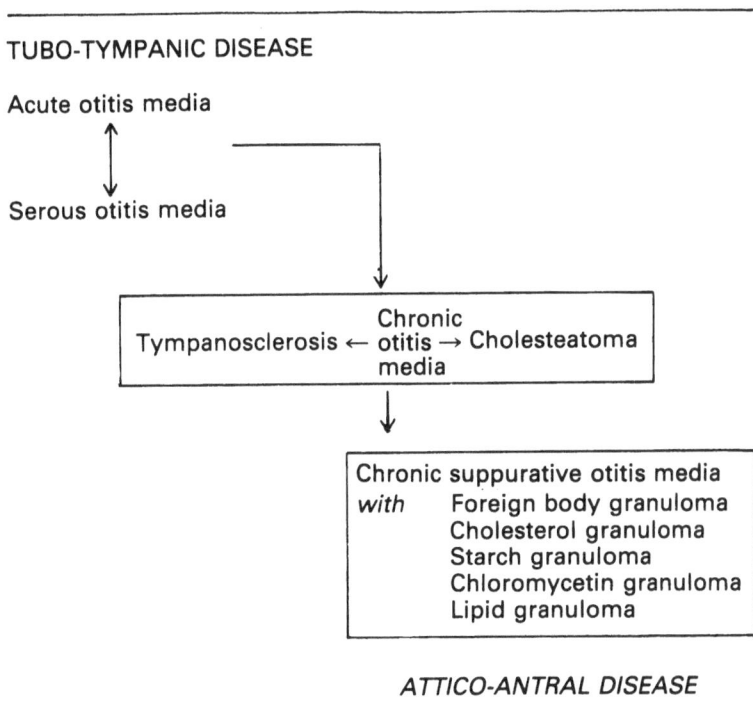

TUBO-TYMPANIC DISEASE

Acute otitis media

Serous otitis media

Tympanosclerosis ← Chronic otitis media → Cholesteatoma

Chronic suppurative otitis media
with   Foreign body granuloma
       Cholesterol granuloma
       Starch granuloma
       Chloromycetin granuloma
       Lipid granuloma

ATTICO-ANTRAL DISEASE

Congenital sensorineural deafness

This may be due to hereditary causes such as a genetic factor, prenatal causes such as abnormal influences on the developing fetus, or perinatal causes, like an accident at or within a few hours of birth.

Hereditary deafness accounts for about one third of all congenital deafness. The Mendelian law determines the transmission of deafness by the dominant or recessive gene. The majority of hereditary deafness, which accounts for about 90%, is transmitted through the recessive gene while the rest is transmitted by the dominant gene.

Two causes of deafness in the prenatal group are the results of maternal infection by rubella and syphilis.

Perinatal causes of deafness are toxaemia of pregnancy in the late stages resulting at times in a premature delivery, trauma at birth or association with anoxia or jaundice.

Hereditary deafness [margin note]

Prenatal causes [margin note]

Table 2.3 What can go wrong in a middle ear infection. The sequelae of a middle ear infection untreated is illustrated in the diagramatic representation of the middle ear and the neighbouring structures

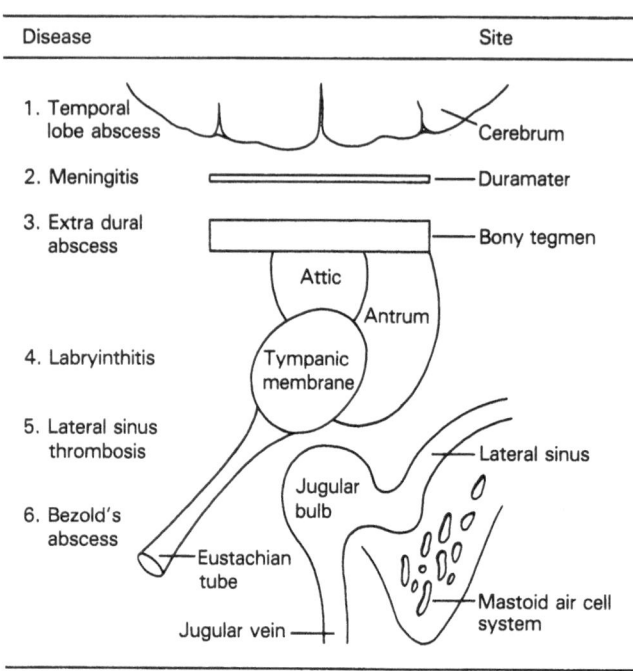

Deafness in childhood

Whatever the congenital cause of sensorineural deafness, it is essential that the affection is detected early in life and the deaf child rehabilitated.

Importance of early diagnosis

For the diagnosis of the deaf child it is very important to bear in mind that the mother of a deaf child is hardly ever wrong. Both subjective and objective hearing tests are preferred in relationship to the history and physical findings to arrive at the diagnosis.

Since two of the main ways the deaf child is rehabilitated are by teaching lip reading and auditory training, it is essential to send the child to the appropriate place for rehabilitation.

Trauma

Acquired sensorineural deafness could be the result of trauma as in:

Head injuries, such as fractures of base of skull and concussion.

Acoustic trauma caused by sound levels of 90 dB or more.

Pressure changes in the middle ear due to high altitude, diving and blast, e.g. bomb.

Infections
Sensorineural deafness may result from any infections such as measles, mumps, chickenpox and meningitis.

Ototoxic drugs
Ototoxic drugs that can cause deafness are aminoglycoside antibiotics, e.g. streptomycin, neomycin, kanamycin and gentamycin, and quinine and cinchona alkaloids, arsenic, lead and mercury.

Ménière's disease

Vertigo
Deafness in this disease is usually unilateral, although about 30% of cases become bilateral. They are first detected due to the crippling vertigo associated with nausea and vomiting. The condition is commonly seen in the age group 35–55 years.

Ménière's disease is also referred to as endolymphatic hydrops, because it is an affection of the membranous labyrinth suspected in 1861 by Ménière and demonstrated in 1938 by Hallpike and Cairns.

Tinnitus
In one half of patients with Ménière's disease the deafness precedes vertigo and in the other, it will accompany the deafness. Hearing improves between attacks, but invariably will lead to a low tone sensorineural loss, progressively getting worse with each attack, always associated with tinnitus. A fullness in the head accompanying these attacks is characteristic and not described in the past.

Acute and chronic phases
Clinically there are two phases, the acute, where the vertigo is the predominant feature, and the chronic where the increasing deafness is more noticeable. The onset of vertigo is always sudden. Very rarely, unconsciousness and diplopia may occur. The duration of vertigo which varies from a few minutes to a few hours is often described as a rotation of himself or of objects about himself.

Audiometry
Diagnosis is supported by audiometry which shows perceptive deafness of a low tone nature with a high tone loss later. Recruitment is present. Speech audiometry shows loss of intelligibility or discrimination out of proportion to the loss of pure tone. The calonic vestibular test shows canal paresis on the affected side.

Ménière's disease should be distinguished from other conditions presenting with mixed deafness and vertigo, such as

Other conditions causing deafness and vertigo
Treatment

acoustic neuroma, epilepsy, labyrinthitis or disseminated and multiple sclerosis.

The treatment is either conservative or surgical (Table 2.2). No surgery should be contemplated until all conservative measures have been tried and the patient finds that the symptoms, especially vertigo are crippling.

Conservative treatment would commence with reassurance and sedation and continue with diet and vasodilator drugs. Avoidance of smoking has helped and irradication of infections like tonsillitis, sinusitis and toothache has played an important part in the management.

Labyrinthitis

Labyrinthitis due either to inflammatory condition as a sequelae of acute or chronic ear disease, or infective conditions secondary to meningitis, can cause perceptive hearing loss.

The history and clinical examination is important to help to arrive at an early diagnosis. Such patients may need hospitalization as they also present with vertigo as a predominant complaint.

Presbycusis

Presbycusis, or senile deafness, is a progressive sensorineural loss with advancing years. It is often bilateral and symmetrical with sex ratio about equal.

Accoustic trauma

Apart from the individual's susceptibility and inherited factors, the exposure to loud noise with acoustic trauma plays an important part in its development.

Hearing aids

Treatment is the use of a hearing aid. There are a large number of postaural aids which cope with different types of sensorineural hearing loss.

Acoustic tumours

These are benign tumours that grow slowly from the sheath of the 8th cranial nerve within the internal auditory meatus.

The first presenting symptom is a sensorineural deafness or tinnitus and is always unilateral. It is very severe when first seen and should *not* be confused with a conductive hearing loss as in otosclerosis.

Recruitment of loudness is very characteristic of sensori-neural deafness. Early examination by the otologist and radio-logical investigation will confirm the diagnosis.

③ The discharging ear

Otitis externa – Subacute otitis media – Chronic otitis media

Discharge from the ear may be from the outer ear or from the middle ear. The outer ear, consisting of skin lining, is liable to

Outer ear   disorders of the skin. The most frequent are infection, such as local boils (furuncles) or more diffuse cellulitis, and inflammation caused by dermatitis or eczema. The middle ear is lined by

Middle ear   mucous membrane and it, too, is liable to infection, as in acute otitis media and inflammation, in serous otitis and chronic otitis media.

Discharge from the middle ear is through a perforation in the ear drum (tympanic membrane) but just as the infection/inflammation spreads outward through the perforation it can also spread internally to adjacent structures.

Otitis externa

Furuncle cellulitis

Prominent features are:

> extreme pain,
> tenderness of outer ear by touching meatus, or pulling ear lobe.
> swelling, redness and occlusion of meatus,
> scanty purulent discharge.

31

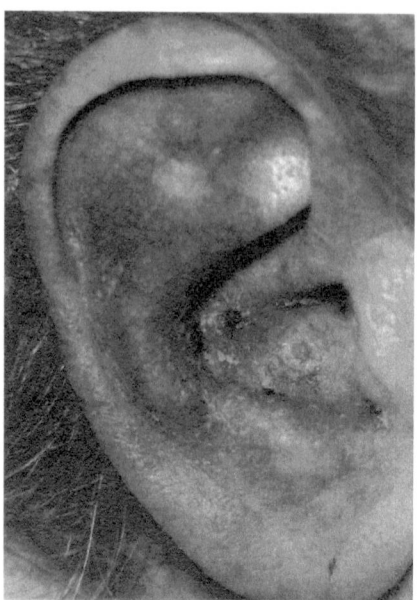

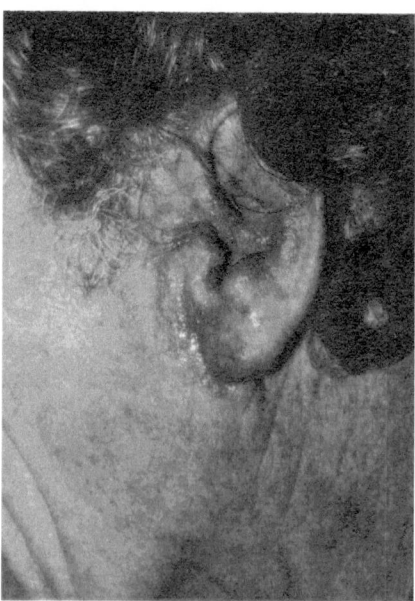

Examples of otitis externa (top) and herpes oticus (bottom) illustrating the difference between the inflammatory disorder of the pinna and external auditory canal

Figure 3.1

Treatment is best by systemic antibiotics by mouth rather than by local measures.

Dermatis and eczema

As in any other acute inflammation of the skin there is swelling, redness, scaling and weeping of the skin lining the external meatus (Figure 3.1). It is primarily an acute inflammation with likely secondary infection by a variety of bacteria or fungi.
Clinical features are:

Clinical
features

watery discharge – thick if infected, may be smelly,
itching,
tenderness,
pain – severe only if secondary infection,
deafness,
generalized redness, scaling, swelling, cracking and discharging lining of external ear,
often bilateral.

Treatment is difficult, not only of the acute phase but because it is a persistent and recurring condition, often associated with tendency to eczema in other areas. *Note* that unilateral otitis externa may be secondary to discharge from the middle ear.
Treatment consists of:

Treatment

Gently cleaning the outer ear to remove debris. This is not easy in practice, because it is time-consuming and demands considerable skills and equipment.

Take swab to identify any specific causal organisms. Often none is detected.

Local applications are popular, usually a mixture of steroid and antibiotic applied as drops or insufflated as a powder. Continual use may lead to sensitization and iatrogenic contact dermatitis.

Cortico-
steroids

Where there is severe pain and local swelling it is justifiable to give a course of antibiotics by mouth to treat likely bacterial infection.

In severe cases with much dermatitis a short course of oral corticosteroids (prednisolone or prednisone) may be dramatically effective.

33

Prevention entails avoiding water and soap, cleaning ears with fingers or buds and scratching.

Acute otitis media (see also Chapter 2)

Discharge in acute otitis media occurs if and when the drum perforates. It usually ceases in a few days and the perforation heals.

Persistent discharge after an acute otitis media may be due to occlusion of the Eustachian tube, by enlarged adenoids or general swelling as part of the upper respiratory infection or, now rarely, from developing mastoiditis.

Clinical features are:

Clinical
features

earache followed by mucopurulent discharge, often blood-stained,
pulsatile discharge through a perforation,
deafness,
discharge sometimes without earache.

Treatment depends on the degree of illness of the child (the condition is rare in adults).

Treatment

If the child is unwell with fever, malaise and pain then a course of antibiotics is indicated (such as ampicillin or amoxycillin).

If the child is well then it is justifiable to wait for a few days as the discharge is quite likely to cease spontaneously.

All children with ear discharge must be followed up to ensure return to normal hearing and normal drum.

Subacute otitis media

In some children discharge may persist for weeks or months after an acute attack. As noted, the most likely causes are continuing infection of nasopharynx and 'glue ear' with thick mucoid discharge. Occlusion of the Eustachian tube by enlarged adenoids may lead to persistent inflammation.

The recommended treatment is:

Treatment

gentle cleansing of outer ear,
local antibiotic drops,

decongestant nasal drops (for short while only), antihistaminics.

If discharge persists then referral is advised to a specialist for examination of the ear under anaesthesia and possible adenoidectomy.

Persistent discharge

Chronic otitis media

The causes of chronic otitis media with ear discharge are not certain. Some may follow an acute infection but many arise without any such attack. The condition is much more frequent in deprived social groups and also has geographical predilections. It is more prevalent in the northern part of Britain than in the south.

There are two types of chronic otitis media with persistent discharge and deafness but without pain.

'Safe' – tubotympanic disease

This type affects the lower parts of the middle ear with a central perforation. There are no risks of spread to adjacent structures. The discharge is from the inflamed mucosa that produces excessive amounts of secretions. It is mucoid and inoffensive and is often associated with blockage of the Eustachian tube.

Blockage of Eustachian tube

Treatment is by referral to a specialist who will examine the ear under an operating microscope and, if pronounced safe, then the aims are to try and dry the ear up by local aural toilet and treating any disorder of the upper respiratory tract.

Treatment

Repair of the damaged drum may be by tympanoplasty.

'Unsafe' – attico-antral disease

This type affects the upper parts of the middle ear – attic antrum. It can erode the ossicles and produces cholesteatoma that can spread and may lead to meningitis and brain abscess.

Cholesteatoma consists of skin that has entered the attic antrum to produce a cyst that becomes infected with erosion of bone.

Cholesteatoma

Perforation in the unsafe ear is peripheral along the bony edge of the middle ear. Granulation tissue and polyps are

35

Smelly discharge   produced and may be seen through the auriscope. Discharge is continuous, scanty and foul smelling (smells of 'cats') as it comes from the infected cholesteatoma.

Surgical treatment   Treatment primarily is to remove the infected and diseased bone and cholesteatoma. This is done surgically. A smooth, wide cavity lined by skin leading to wide, external canal is achieved.

Long-term follow-up   Long-term follow-up is necessary to ensure that the cavity remains clean and free of debris. Deafness is inevitable. Once the cavity is lined by skin, discharge will only occur from inflammation from accumulated debris or from incomplete eradication of the disease.

4 Vertigo

Physiological and pathological vertigo – Peripheral and central vertigo – Clinical assessment

Vertigo is a false sense of movement either of the patient himself (subjective) or of his surroundings (objective).

Vertigo may sometimes be so severe as to affect the autonomic system such that the patient may present with pallor, sweating and may vomit and even fall to the ground.

Vertigo is caused by an abnormal stimulation from outside applied to any of the sense organs concerned in the maintenance of equilibrium or by disease of these sensory end organs and their central connections.

Physiological and patholigical vertigo

Physiological   Physiological vertigo is due to no fault in the human body but to unusual stimulation of the normal structures, for example giddiness due to heights or motion of spinning round.

Pathological   Patholigical vertigo is due to disease of organs or structure responsible for maintaining equilibrium. This group includes affections to other functions used in balance, i.e. diplopia, blindness and motor neuron disease.

37

Peripheral and central vertigo

Another way of classifying vertigo is by the site of the lesion.

Peripheral When it arises from conditions outside the brain, it is termed peripheral as opposed to central vertigo caused by lesions within the brain.

Central vertigo is often associated with a disturbance of one or more of the following structures:

Central the vestibular system of the inner ear, i.e. semi-circular canals,
vestibular division of the 8th cranial nerve,
vestibular nucleus in the brain stem,
disruption of the pathway between vestibular nuclei and the cortex of the temporal lobe,
cerebellum.

Clinical assessment

When a patient presents with vertigo it is necessary to ascertain if the cause is related to the ear and if associated with tinnitus and deafness and whether there is pathology, primarily, arising from the ear.

Diagnosis may be obvious but to arrive at the cause of vertigo it is important to obtain a clear history. Questions should include:

History onset of first attack,
relationship to position in space, not only of the whole body but head in relation to the body,
details of past medical history including habits,
pattern of attack.

Clinical examination should not only include routine ENT
Examinations examination but also neurological examination.

The investigation for vestibular dysfunction should always be preceded by tests to exclude metabolic disorders such as anaemia and thyroid dysfunction if indicated.

Vestibular analysis includes simple audiometric tests fol-
Vestibular lowed by caloric tests and electronystagmography. Other
analysis special tests are only available in certain special units.

Radiological investigations for vertigo follow from the history and ENT examination.

Sinuses – Eustachian tube dysfunction, secondary to sinus

Radiological
investigations
 infection or pathology in postnasal spaces.

Mastoids and temporal bones – chronic suppurative otitis media.

Tomogram of internal auditory meatus – pathology in internal auditory meatus like acoustic neuroma.

Cervical spine – basilar vertebral insufficiency.

Brain scan
 Following X-ray, a patient may need a brain scan if there is an indication to exclude a pathology in the brain.

A summary of the causes of vertigo is shown in Table 4.1.

Table 4.1 Summary of causes of vertigo

Outer ear	Middle ear	Inner ear	Brain
1. Wax	1. Barotraumatic otitis media	1. Méniéres disease	1. Acoustic neuroma
2. Trauma to tympanic membrane	2. Caisson disease	2. Otosclerosis	2. Menigintis
3. Fractured skull – temporal bone	3. Glomus jugular tumour	3. Perceptive deafness	3. Epilepsy
	4. Otosclerosis	4. Labyrinthitis	4. Temporal lobe abscess
	5. Carcinoma of middle ear	5. Drug toxicity quinine streptomycin	5. Anoxia of brain
	6. Chronic supperative otitis media	6. Syphilis	6. Ramsay Hunt Syndrome
	7. Fractured temporal bone	7. Vertibuloneuronitis	
	8. Serous otitis media due to Eustachian tube dysfunction	8. Acoustic trauma	

5 Tinnitus

Tinnitus is the hearing of sounds without any evident external cause. Tinnitus may be intermittent as in the case of an acoustic neuroma or continous as in a case of a benign aural disease or with no evidence of disease at all.

Two physiopathological groups can be separated. The first group is objective tinnitus when the symptom is audible to the patient and the clinician. The causes can be:

Objective tinnitus

Causes

foreign body in external auditory canal,
mandibular joint dysfunction as in Costen's syndrome,
tensor tympani disorder after facial palsy,
respiratory tinnitus due to patulous Eustachian tube,
vascular tinnitus, glomus tumour, arteriovenous
aneurysms.

Subjective tinnitus is more common and is further divided into two groups, namely central and peripheral, according to whether it could be masked. Sectioning the 8th cranial nerve need not necessarily abolish tinnitus.

Subjective tinnitus

Clinical groups

Two clinical forms of tinnitus are those with or without deafness.

41

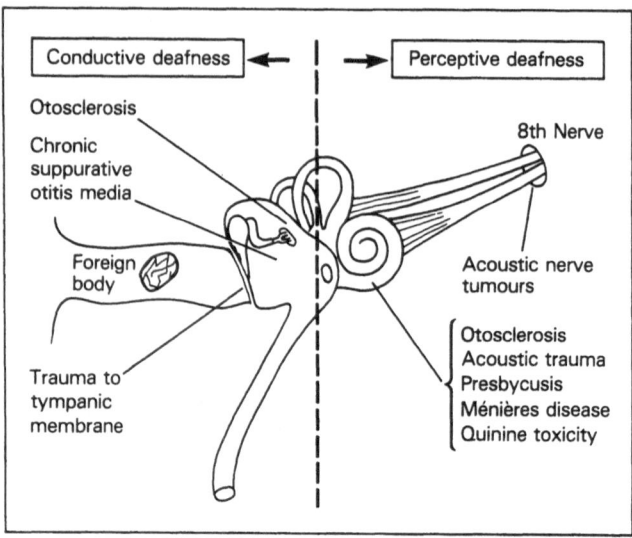

Figure 5.1	Causes of tinnitus

With deafness

Those with a conductive hearing loss have low tone and intermittent noises. Those with perceptive hearing loss have high tone continuous noises. Conditions presenting with deafness and tinnitus are shown in Figure 5.1.

Without deafness

Though no cause may be found it is essential to exclude extra-aural causes such as:

Oral pathology, i.e. impacted wisdom teeth, apical abscess and neoplasms of the nasopharynx.

Metabolic disorder, i.e. anaemia and thyrotoxicosis.

Cerebrovascular abnormality and intracranial tumours.

Management

In tinnitus management is more important than treatment. This is because successful treatment is not often posssible. In the great majority of cases of tinnitus it is likely to persist either for ever or cease spontaneously for no good reason.

It is wrong and untrue to suggest to the patient with tinnitus that it can be cured by medical or surgical treatments. Rather it is better to state honestly that it may be permanent, but some optimism is appropriate for those cases that may cease naturally.

There is no effective surgical treatment for tinnitus *per se*. Relief may result from sedatives and antidepressant drugs.

No satis-
factory
treatment

Facial paralysis

*Upper motor neuron paralysis – Lower motor neuron paralysis
– Ascertainment of level of lesion – Management of facial palsy*

The inability of a muscle or a group of muscles of the face to contract, usually as a result of damage to motor neurons, although it can occur due to interference at the neuromuscular function, is commonly referred to as facial paralysis.

The nucleus of the facial nerve lies deep in the substance of the pons. The upper motor neuron fibres of the facial nerve originate in the opposite cortex and any disruption of this nerve pathway resulting in facial weakness is an upper motor neuron paralysis of the facial nerve.

Upper motor neuron paralysis

This varies greatly in degree but the essential features are as follows:

Paralysis is obvious but weakness is incomplete.

The lower part of the face is affected most.

Though there is no wasting of muscles, they are more rigid than normal.

Features

After a variable interval of time the return of function of

45

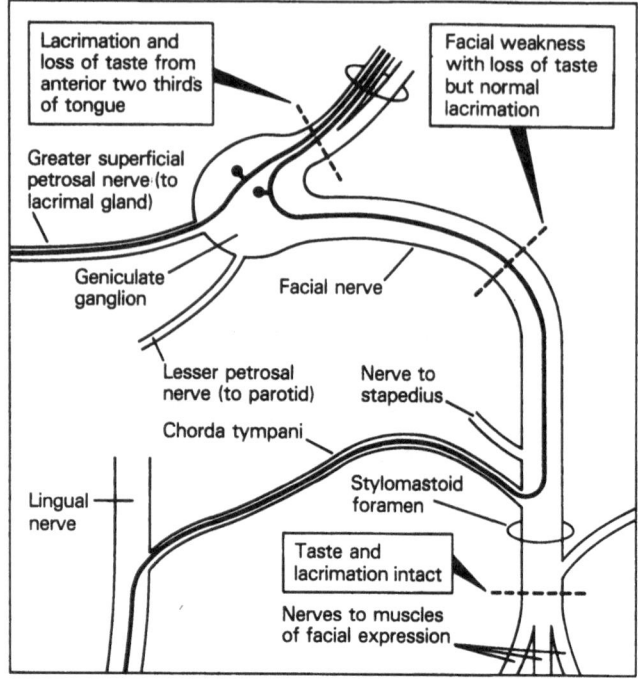

Diagram of the facial nerve showing how degree of paralysis depends upon the site of the lesion

Figure 6.1

facial muscles is greater and quicker in the upper part of the face than the lower part and recovery more complete than the accompanying paralysis of limbs of the same side.

Lower motor neuron paralysis

Lower motor neuron paralysis of the face is characterized by the weakness being distributed equally between the upper and lower parts of the face. The other obvious features are:

The face is asymmetrical at rest.

Lower eye lid and angle of mouth sag on affected side.

Features

Tears overflow and saliva may dribble out on the affected side.

Mouth is pulled to active side on smiling.

46

Food may collect in the cheek due to the paralysed buccinator.

There is a lack of tone and wasting of muscles.

Pathway of facial nerve

The site of a lesion in the lower motor neuron paralysis could be anywhere between the site of the nucleus in the pons to the exit of the facial nerve at the stylomastoid foramen. The facial nerve as it leaves the pons traverses the cerebropontine angle to enter the internal auditory meatus accompanied by the nervus intermedius and the cochlear and vestibular division of the eighth cranial nerve. The facial nerve is in close proximity to the structures of the middle ear in its intrapetrous part of the course until it emerges at the stylomastoid foramen as illustrated in Figure 6.2.

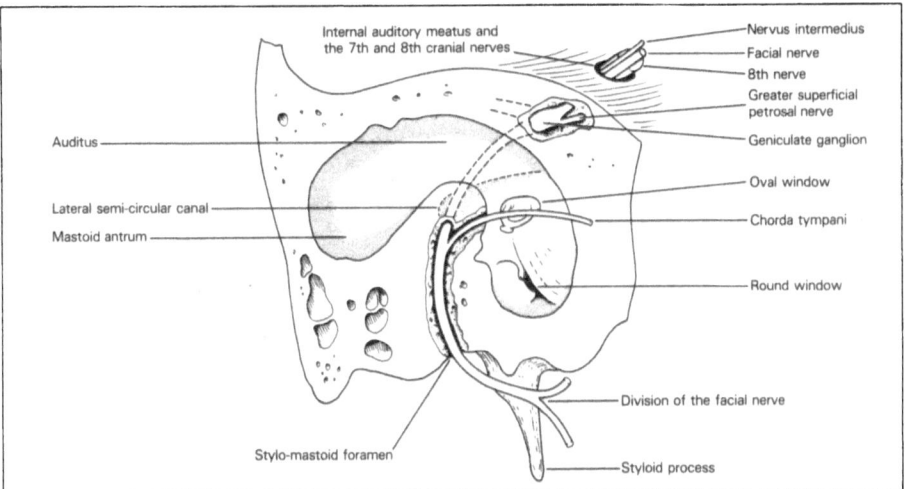

A view of the infranuclear course of the facial nerve as it traverses the temporal bone to show its close proximity to the middle ear structures

Figure 6.2

Ascertainment of level of lesion

Having ascertained that a facial nerve palsy is either upper motor neuron or lower motor neuron it is essential to determine the level of the lesion to understand the exact clinical picture.

Various tests to illustrate the absence or presence of a

Table 6.1 Site of lesion of the facial nerve and the tests in relation to symptoms and signs

Anatomical site	Symptom or sign in addition to facial paralysis	Tests
Internal auditory meatus	Vertigo, deafness	Electronystagmograph Caloric tests. Audiometry
Tympano-mastoid course	Hyperacusis stapedius muscle paralysed.	Absent stapedial reflex on impedance measurement
	Loss of taste due to chorda tympani being affected	Test with salt and sugar and/or salivation
Extracranial course	Paralysis of facial muscles	Electromyography

Tests function of the facial nerve determine the level of the lesion as shown in Table 6.1 and help to determine the causes of peripheral facial paralysis in relation to anatomical sites, as shown in Table 6.2.

Table 6.2 Causes of peripheral facial paralysis in relation to anatomical sites

Anatomical site	Cause
Intracranial	Tumours Vascular accident ⎱ Poliomyelitis ⎰ Brain stem lesions Multiple sclerosis
Intratemporal	Bell's palsy Herpes oticus – Ramsey Hunt syndrome Otitis media – acute and chronic Tumours – Glomus tympanicum Trauma – RTA and surgery
Infratemporal	Parotid tumours Trauma – RTA and surgery
Miscellaneous	Sarcoidosis Leukaemia Infective mononucleosis Polyneuritis

Children In children there are different varieties of causes and hence one should not assume it is a Bell's palsy. If the palsy was present at birth it is very important to differentiate between congenital and traumatic as illustrated in Table 6.3.

Table 6.3 Differences between congenital and traumatic palsy in children

	Congenital	*Traumatic*
History	Family history of facial and/or other anomalies No recovery of facial function after birth	Though total paralysis noted, some recovery later
Clinical examination	Other congenital anomalies present, Palsy limited to lower lip or upper face	Haemotympanum Ecchymosis Tics
X-ray finding	Anomalies involving external, middle or inner ear	Fracture of skull involving temporal bone
Electro-myography	Reduced or absent response. No evidence of degeneration	Normal at birth and then loss of spontaneous units followed by fibrillation

Management of facial palsy

In every case, when determining the type of facial paralysis, the nature and prognosis should be explained to the patient with the appropriate reassurance.

Once the clinical diagnosis has been made the patient may either be treated at home as in cases of idiopathic facial palsy – Bell's palsy, or hospitalized for surgical intervention or management of general medical state as in a stroke.

Care of eye In all cases, the care of the eye to prevent corneal abrasion is important. Initially use chloromycetin eye drops and in later stages use tarsorrhaphy.

Care of mouth The sagging cheek and corner of the mouth could be supported and the patient can be taught self-massage of the paralysed muscles.

The use of steroids is debatable in idiopathic facial palsy.

Steroids
Decompres-
sion of facial
nerve

The author does not use steroids but will consider decompression of the facial nerve if there is no recovery in 4–6 weeks after onset of paralysis.

When in doubt about the nature of the palsy and its management it is advisable to consult an otolaryngologist.

7 Anosmia

*Anatomy and physiology of sensation of smell and taste –
Causes of anosmia – Clinical assessment – treatment – Course
and outcome*

Anosmia implies complete loss of sense of smell. Often it is
accompanied by loss of taste. In addition there are other
subjective disorders of smell.

Anosmia – complete loss of smell
Hyposmia – partial loss of smell
Cacosmia – perception of bad smell
Parosmia – sensation of non-existent smells

Anatomy and physiology of sensation of smell and taste

Figure 7.1 illustrates the nervous connections that are involved in olfactory and taste sensation.

Causes of anosmia

The causes of anosmia may be:
Nasal obstruction due to a foreign body, polyps or deviated
septum,

51

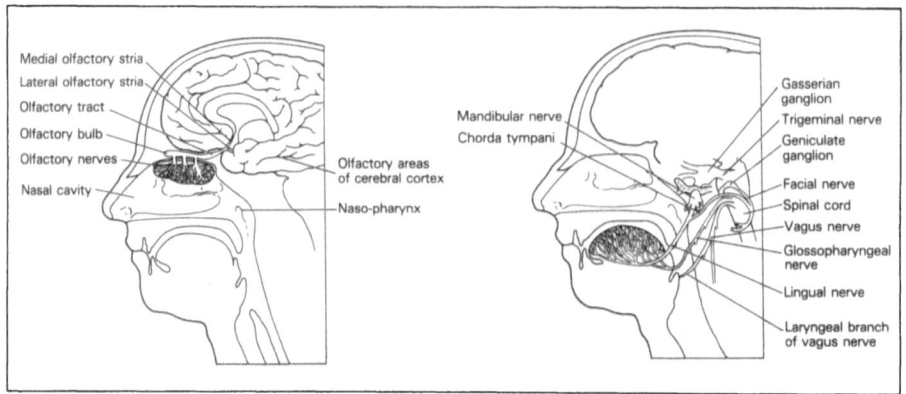

The nervous connections that are involved in olfactory and taste sensation

Figure 7.1

allergic rhinitis,
atrophic rhinitis,
peripheral neuritis,
trauma,
intracranial lesion,
industrial hazards,
unknown.

Clinical assessment

The following facts about the history should be ascertained.

Was the speed of onset sudden, e.g. a foreign body, or slow, e.g. a slow growing tumour?

Is there any taste involvement and is the olfactory involvement intracranial or extracranial?

Are there any precipitating factors, such as upper respiratory infections or specific fevers?

History

Are there any other illnesses such as meningitis or cerebrovascular accident?

Is there a family history or a past history of allergies?

Has a trauma occurred such as a road traffic accident, a boxing injury or past surgery to nose?

Are there occupational hazards involved such as noxious chemical fumes?

The following examinations should be made.

Hold a mirror under nose with shut mouth to note degree of misting.

Whether nasal obstruction is bilateral or unilateral and if so the side.

Inspect nose with speculum and with good light for foreign bodies, polyps, deviated septum or rhinitis.

Examinations

Examine mouth and note movements of soft palate as a sign of intracranial lesion.

Check dental state to exclude infection, especially dental cyst, apical abscess or even an ora-antral fistula.

Examine ears for serous otitis. Secondary to nasopharyngeal pathology, i.e. Eustachian tube obstruction.

Examine C V S hypertension causing recurrent nose bleeds.

Examine C N S to exclude intracranial lesion.

Treatment

Ascertain the possible causes and decide on referral to specialist care or by general practitioner.

Referral to specialist

foreign bodies,
trauma to exclude fractures and possible CSF rhinorrhoea, and for medicolegal reasons,
polyps for removal.

Care by general practitioner

Allergic rhinitis can be treated by antihistamines, local steroid inhalation or local cromoglycate inhalation. If there is no improvement refer to a specialist for possible desensitization or submucous diathermy.

Course and outcome

The outcome of anosmia is related to its causes. Serious specific causes are uncommon, i.e. tumours or neurological disorders or trauma.

Common causes are upper respiratory infections, and allergic or atrophic rhinitis. Many of these will resolve naturally in time with return of sensation of smell.

Note the significance of presenting symptoms related to outcomes.

	'doctor, I can't breathe'	nasal obstruction due to rhinitis, polyps or foreign body
	'runny nose'	Allergic rhinitis or foreign body
	'postnasal drip'	nasal polyps and sinus infection
Symptoms related to outcomes	'bleeding from nose'	foreign body, tumour
	'headache'	sinus infection, trauma, intracranial tumour
	'double vision'	intracranial causes
	'red eyes'	ethmoidal pathology (infection, tumour)
	'can't taste'	can't taste without smell, therefore no stimulus to olfactory area.

Nasal obstruction and nasal discharge

Nasal obstruction – Nasal discharge

Nasal obstruction and discharge are frequent symptoms. The extent of their discomfort and disability depends on subjective and objective factors.

Some persons with severe symptoms may have few detectable abnormalities and some with gross abnormalities may not complain of nasal obstruction or discharge.

It has to be honestly stated that the nature and causes in many cases are difficult to define and hence management is often incompletely successful.

Nasal obstruction

Nasal obstruction may result from an obvious mechanical cause with a restricted airway or as a sensation of 'nasal blockage' with a good airway.

Nasal obstruction in children is almost always due to a mechanical cause, but many may not complain because of the ability of mouth breathing to overcome the blocked nasal airways.

In adults a clear mechanical cause may not be found and speculation as to the possible aetiology may be unproductive.

55

Causes of persistent nasal obstruction

Acute and
transient

Persistent

Acute and transient nasal obstruction are almost always the result of acute viral infections, are self-limiting and do not require specific treatment. Persistent (chronic) nasal obstruction has different causes in children and adults. In children it can be caused by

Children

grossly enlarged adenoids,
vasomotor rhinitis, possibly allergic, atrophic or idiopathic,
   arising from
      foreign body (rare),
      congenital choanal atresia (very rare),
      nasal and postnasal tumours (very, very rare).

In adults persistent nasal obstruction can be caused by:

Adults

deviated nasal septum
   (present in one quarter of all adults),
vasomotor rhinitis, idopathic or allergic,
chronic sinusitis,
nasal polyps,
iatrogenic, from excessive use of vasoconstrictive
   nasal preparations with rebound vasodilation,
after repeated nasal surgery for nasal and postnasal tumours
   (very rare).

Effects

In adults the effects are chronic pharyngitis and laryngitis, snoring and gum disorders.

In children the effects are speech distortion, hearing loss, cough and snoring.

Clinical assessment

Enquiries should be made about the history:

History

when first noted,
aggravating or relieving factors,
associated symptoms,
smoking history,
dogs, cats or other animal contacts.

In *children* further questions on the following should be asked:

Children

snoring,
runny nose,
thick catarrh,
nose bleeds,
cough,
earaches,
deafness,
possibility of foreign body insertion,
general health,
smoking in family,
pets.

Any history of trauma, headaches, malaise, or purulent nasal discharge should be inquired about and the state of consciousness established.

The *child* should be examined for:

Examinations

visual acuity,
eyelids – movement, swelling,
eyeball movements,
facial deformity,
nose and nasal discharge,
neck stiffness.

Further tests should be made if necessary such as sinus X-rays and a blood picture.

Adults question should be asked the following:

History in
adults

sort of nasal discharge,
nose bleeds,
sense of smell,
headaches,
previous surgery or trauma,
cough,
smoking history,
hobbies and pets.

Examinations

Anosmia

An examination of the nose and throat should be made and a mirror test is useful to assess degrees of nasal obstruction. Anosmia (see Chapter 7) should be looked for and other possible causes should be noted such as atrophic rhinitis, neuronitis of cranial nerve I or *rarities* such as TB, syphilis, rhinoscleroma, neoplasm, fungal infection or intracranial neoplasm.

Treatment

In children the following treatments should be considered.

remove adenoids (for better nasal airway and to prevent Eustachian tube obstruction),

remove foreign body,

for vasomotor rhinitis

Vasomotor
rhinitis

   antihistaminics (trial)
   avoidance of allergens
   possibly desensitization
   submucous diathermy
   avoid long-term vasoconstrictor applications.

In adults treatment consists of:

for vasomotor rhinitis
   antihistaminics (trial)
   removal of polyps
   submucous diathermy,
for deviated nasal septum
   submucous resection (SMR) (To improve airway, aid free flow of mucus and keep all ostia opening into nasal

Deviated nasal
septum

cavity patent).

Nasal discharge

Some nasal discharge is normal and essential for normal respiration.

Excessive nasal discharge can lead to one or more of the following:

nasal obstruction,
epiphora (eye watering),

Effects

epistaxis,
headache,
anosmia,
diplopia.

Postnasal discharge is a distinct type, usually associated with the more 'posterior' discharge. The indications are: antrochoanal polyp or carcinoma of nasopharynx (Figures 8.1 and 8.2). It can produce:

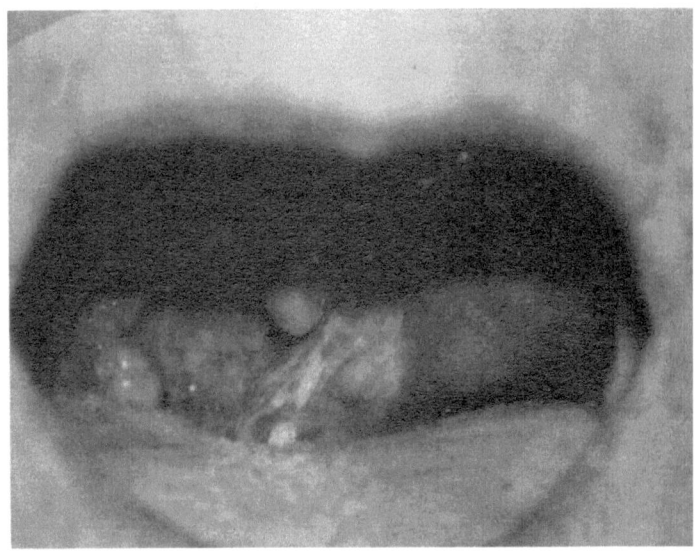

Carcinoma of the tonsil

Figure 8.1

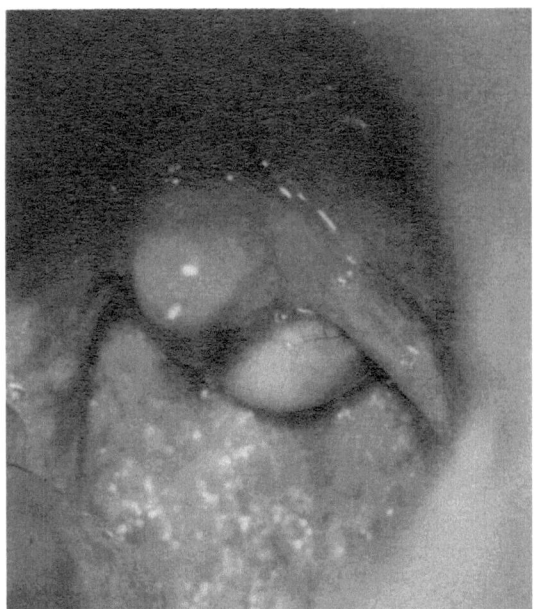

Antro-chonanal polyp

Figure 8.2

Postnasal
discharge
    sore throat,
    hoarseness,
    cough,
    stridor,
    breathlessness.
    Loss of taste and smell. Indications for these are chronic maxillary sinus infection, nasal polyps.

Causes

The nature of nasal discharge can point to possible causes. If it is seromucoid, it can be caused by:

Seromucoid
    common cold,
    vasomotor rhinitis,
    sinusitis,
    enlarged adenoids.

If the discharge is bloody, it can be caused by:

Bloody
    foreign body,
    trauma,
    postsurgery,
    neoplasms, either benign or malignant.

⑨ Nose bleeds

Age–sex distribution – Sites of nose bleedings – Causes – associated symptoms – Management

Bleeding from the nose is a common 'emergency'. In any year in a general practice 2500 persons there are likely to occur 5–10 nose bleeds of sufficient severity to require medical attention.

Age–sex distribution

Nose bleeds are more frequent in males. The age prevalence peaks at 10–20 years and again at 60–70+ years. The reasons for this are uncertain. In youth there may be physiological factors and in the elderly nose bleeds may be related to inevitable atherosclerotic changes.

Sites of nose bleeding

Anterior bleeding

It is important in practice to differentiate the sites of bleed (Figure 9.1). Bleeds may be anterior or posterior, high or low, and septal or lateral. Anterior bleeding occurs in 80–90% of cases. Low bleeds come from Little's area (Figure 9.1) and high bleeds from the anterior ethmoidal artery. Posterior bleeding is

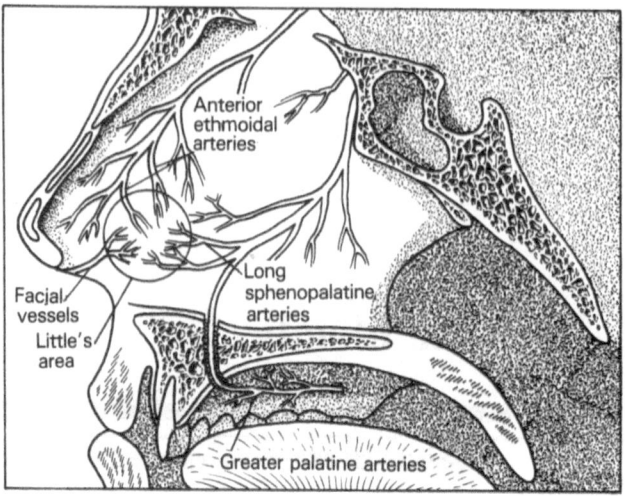

Sites of nose bleeds

Figure 9.1

Posterior bleeding
rare and comes from the posterior ethmoidal (high) or internal maxillary (low arteries).

Causes

In most cases (over 80%) of nose bleeding no definite cause is found. Specific causes may be:

nasal or sinus infections,
nasal allergy,
trauma to nose,
high blood pressure – although frequently found in elderly persons with nose bleeds it is rarely the actual cause,
blood diseases,
familial telangiectasia,
renal or liver failure.

Associated symptoms

Check the following symptoms for significance.

A headache may indicate that the nose bleeding is related to hypertension.

If there is a cough, check if there is posterior bleed, if there is a clot in postnasal space, or if aspiration of blood is occurring.

Nausea may be caused by swallowed blood or vertigo.

A sore throat may be caused by infection.

If the patient feels 'faint', the reason could be vasovagal or it could be caused by shock from blood loss.

If the patient complains of tinnitus he could be anaemic or thyrotoxic.

Management

An assessment should be made of the effects of blood loss and whether a transfusion is necessary. Identify the source and cause of the bleeding and apply methods to stop the bleeding:

Sit the patient up over a bowl.

Pinch the nose.

Conservative

Apply ice packs to the nose.

Ask the patient to blow nose to clear out clots.

Examine the nose and general condition.

In four out of five patients bleeding stops within 1–2 hours. If bleeding continues, in the case of an anterior bleed, pack the nose and cauterize. For a posterior bleed, pack the nose. If bleed still continues, refer the patient to a specialist in hospital.

Continued bleeding

10 Epiphora

Causes – Clinical assessment – Treatment – Practical points

Epiphora is an excessive watering of the eyes due to inadequate drainage of tears down the tear (lacrimal) ducts. It results from obstruction of the lacrimal duct.

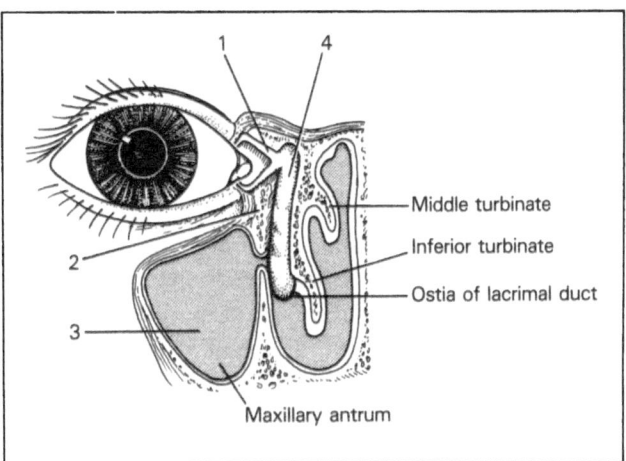

Diagram to illustrate the relationship between the lacrymal sac and neighbouring structures. (1) common site of infection, including fungal; (2) when sac wall is involved due to any cause it will give rise to dacryocystitis; (3) tumours of the maxillary antrum will not only give rise to diplopia but also epiphora; (4) tumours of lacrymal sac are very rare

Figure 10.1

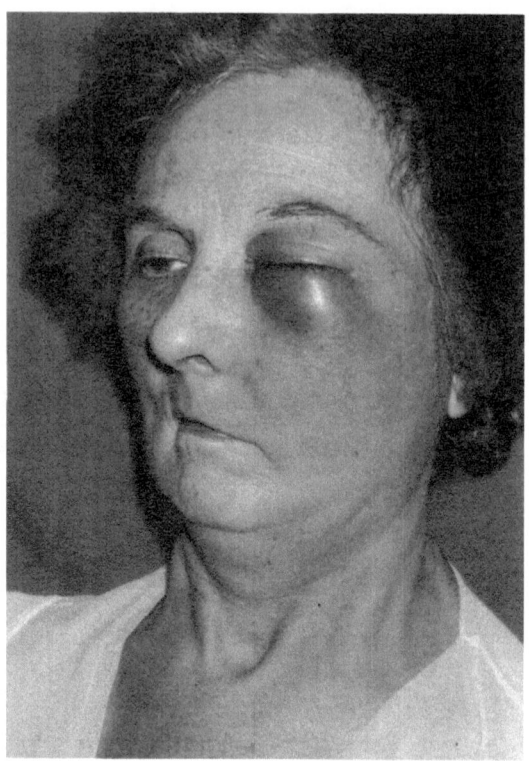

Patient with carcinoma of the maxillary antrum which produces nasolacrymal duct obstruction

Figure 10.2

Causes

Congenital 'delayed development' obstruction of the tear ducts in newborn babies leads to sticky eyes and watering. It is the most frequent cause of the 'sticky eye'. Sticky eye usually is caused by drying of mucus in the tear and not to infection.

'Sticky' eye   Antibiotic drops or ointments are not necessary and surgical interference, such as probing, should be resisted until the ducts have had time to enlarge and develop naturally. This may take 6 months or more.

Foreign bodies, infection (blepharitis) or ectropion cause narrowing (stenosis) of lacrimal duct.

Nasal polypi, allergic rhinitis, and benign or malignant tumours of nose or sinuses cause obstruction of the nasal section of the lacrimal duct (Figure 10.2).

Facial injuries occurring in sport, road accidents or assault causing fractures of nasal bones.

Dacryocystitis, an infection of the lacrimal duct, causes narrowing, swelling and purulent discharge from the punctum.

Facial paralysis, a weakness of the muscles of the eyelids, leads to loss of pumping action and eversion of eyelid and occlusion of punctum and duct.

Trigeminal neuralgia probably causes reflex excessive tear production.

Clinical assessment

In cases of epiphora check for:

redness of eye,
tender swelling along the lacrimal duct,
unilateral mucopurulent nasal discharge and nasal obstruction.
headaches and blurred vision, due to the eye watering and excess mucus, possible causes, such as trauma, infection, allergy, and facial paralysis.

To exclude sinus infection and possible causal organisms, the following investigations should be made.

Investigations

Sinus X-rays (Figure 10.3).
Full blood picture and ESR.
Nasal swab for bacteriology.
Specialists may try to dilate the punctum and wash through the lacrimal duct to test patency.

Treatment

Many of the causes of epiphora may resolve naturally, therefore over-enthusiastic radical treatments should be delayed unless there are urgent indications such as acute abscess formation in the duct or possible tumours.

In most cases the patient, or parents, should receive a clear explanation of the nature and likely course and outcome, emphasizing the likelihood of natural spontaneous resolution.

Local measures include bathing the eye and possible use of
Antibiotics   antibiotic eye drops for short periods. For nasal obstruction due

67

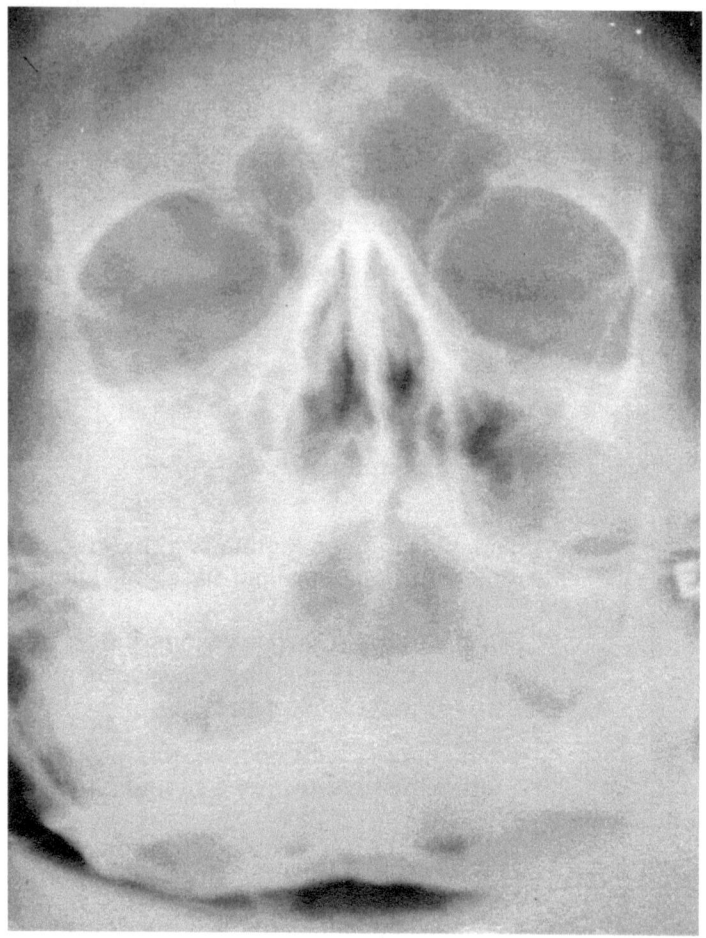

Figure 10.3

Sinus X-ray showing opaque antrum due to carcinoma causing naso-lacrimal duct obstruction

to allergies or congestion, decongestant drops and inhalations may help. Systemic antiobiotics may be necessary for acute dacryocystitis.

Practical points

Sticky watering eyes in infants tend to get better spontaneously given time.

In adults treatment is based on causes.

Some cases will require advice from an ophthalmic surgeon,

others from an ENT surgeon.

Radical measures are indicated only after adequate trial of simple local measures.

Urgent referral is necessary if severe infection is unresponsive to antibiotics and if tumours are considered as possible cause.

11 Sore throat

Who gets them and when – Causes – Inter-relations – Clinical types – Lymphoid changes

Sore throat is a frequent symptom. In a practice of 2500 patients 50–100 will consult annually for 'sore throat'.

Sore throat can be the presentation of a range of conditions, from minor transient infections to lethal neoplasms or blood diseases.

Although the common causes are minor, safe and self-limiting, in any unusual sore throat that does not resolve within a couple of weeks, if the patient is more severely ill than may be expected or if there are unusual associated features such as voice changes and breathlessness, then beware of sinister dangerous possibilities.

Who gets them and when?

Sore throats are predominantly conditions of children and adolescents. It is likely that there are underlying natural immunological changes that relate to this pattern of prevalence. Beware of 'sore throats' in the very young and the old. The young (under 3) do not complain of 'sore throat' – their mothers do so for them. The condition may be 'croup', epiglottitis, retropharyngeal abscess or even diphtheria. The old do not

'Sore throats' in young children

71

Old people suffer from ordinary sore throat. Tonsillitis is unusual and the soreness may result from chronic local irritation, association with chronic chest conditions or neoplasia.

Causes

Bacterial infections

Definable bacterial infections, predominantly *Strep. haemolyticus* are found in less than one half of patients. Other causal organisms may be *Strep. pneumoniae* and *H. influenzae*. Gonococcal, syphilitic and diphtherial infections are extremely rare and are unlikely to be encountered in a general practitioner's professional lifetime.

Glandular fever

In 10% or so the sore throat may be part of infectious mononucleosis (glandular fever) or rarities such as leukaemia, agranulocytosis, and new growths.

No definable cause

In 45% no definable cause can be found. There are various suggested possibilities such as viruses, smoking, alcohol, sinus infection, nasal allergies and other causes of nasal obstruction.

Inter-relations

Sore throat cannot be considered as an isolated condition. The throat is but a part of the respiratory tract – related to nose, sinuses, larynx, bronchi and lungs. The possible relationships are shown in Table 11.1.

Clinical types

Clinically and practically the normal 'throat' comprises the pharynx, tonsils and cervical glands.

Acute tonsillitis

This is a local infection of the tonsils and glands plus variable degrees of systemic reactions, such as fever, rash and other effects. Exact aetiological diagnosis is not possible. It is likely that less than one half is caused by *Strep. haemolyticus*.

Treatment

Treatment must be empirical. 'Mild' cases with little local or systemic disturbances do not require specific therapy with antibiotics. Those more severely disturbed should be treated

Table 11.1 Interrelationship of symptoms and signs and sequelae if not resolved

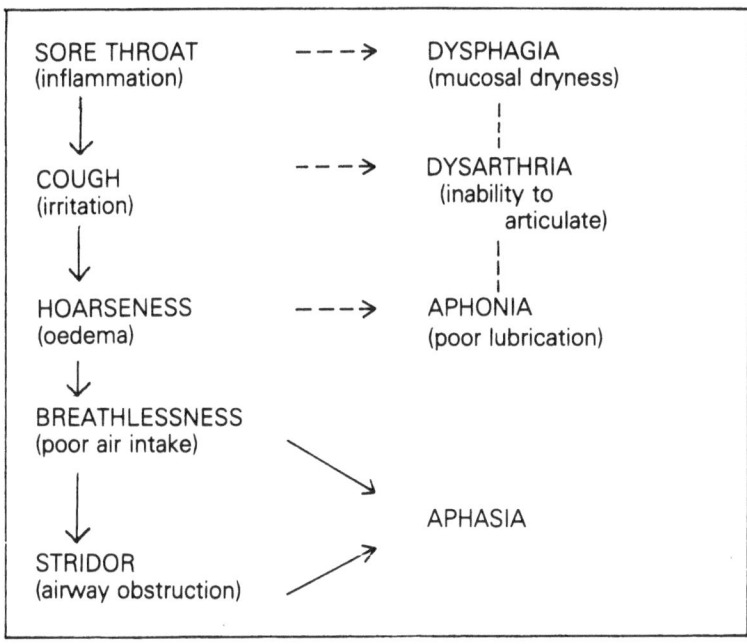

with penicillin, either by injection or oral medication.

Quinsy

This is a peritonsillar cellulitis that may lead to abscess. It is caused by *Strep. haemolyticus* and it should be treated with penicillin by injection (because oral medication is painfully difficult or impossible). Surgical incision should be necessary only rarely.

Acute pharyngitis

This is part of a more general inflammation of the upper respiratory tract with cough, nasal discharge and hoarseness, probably caused by viruses. Treatment is by nonspecific measures to relieve symptoms.

Laryngitis

Laryngitis produces hoarseness, cough and stridor. It is caused by viruses and treatment is non-specific.

Epiglottitis

Epiglottitis is very rare, but the inflammatory process demands urgent hospitalization. It is caused by *H. influenzae*. Treatment is with ampicillin and or chloramphemicol and steroids and humidification to help improve airway.

Cervical adenitis

This may be more prominent than the throat infection. Cervical glands are palpable in all children and are part of a natural enlargement of all lymphoid tissues. Palpability does not necessarily mean infection or disease.

Chronic pharyngitis

This is the term given to a persistent soreness of the throat. It is often associated with:

   smoking,
   alcohol,
   talking,
   nasal obstruction,
   paranasal sinus infection.

Malignant tumours

Malignant tumours of the tonsils or postnasal space can cause 'soreness' of the throat but abnormal appearances soon lead to likely diagnosis.

Lymphoid changes

Tonsils, adenoids and cervical glands change in size naturally at various ages (Figure 11.1). Tonsils are small in infancy and at their largest at 3–8 years. A secondary increase in tonsillar

Sore throat

size occurs in some teenagers and then tonsillar shrinkage occurs from the teens onwards. They are small and atrophic in the elderly.

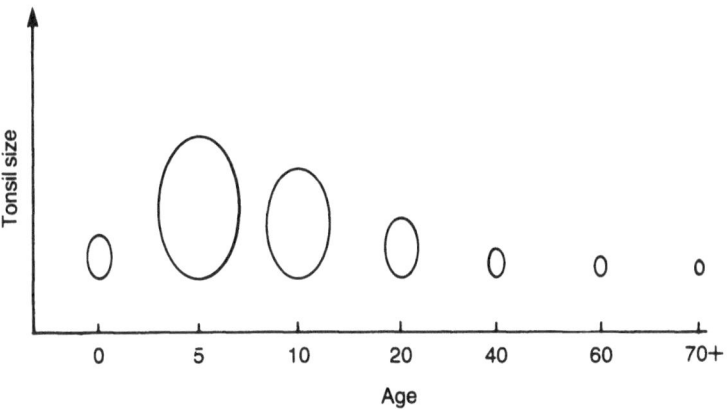

Diagram to show the relative size of tonsils with age

Figure 11.1

12 Hoarseness and stridor

Children – Adults – Aphasia – Dysarthria

Hoarseness may be acute (inflammatory) or chronic (neoplastic or neurological) and leads to an unnatural deepening of the voice with a harsh quality instead of being sharp and crisp.

Hoarseness and stridor, usually accompanied by some cough and breathlessness are features of some laryngeal disorder. Sometimes there are associated symptoms such as fever, weight loss – possibly neoplastic, earache from referred pain, a mass in the neck from secondary deposits and anxiety and depression.

Associated symptoms

The larynx is a relatively small and finely structured organ designed for speech and breathing. Minor pathological changes can lead to major effects.

The most frequent causes of laryngeal disease in practice are, in order:

Causes of laryngeal disease

infections,
misuse,
trauma,
neoplasms,
congenital malformations,
foreign bodies.

Swelling and obstruction of the small larynx in children are potentially more dangerous than in adults.

All cases of stridor and hoarseness must be treated with

respect because, whilst the majority of cases are relatively minor, benign and self-limiting, the same symptoms may be the forerunners of dangerous and life-threatening diseases. The effects of major disorders may be catastrophically rapid or insidiously progressive.

Children

Hoarseness and stridor in children can be caused by neonatal defects, croup, epiglottitis, a foreign body, papillomata, diphtheria or a neoplasm.

Neonatal

Stridor in the neonate may range from noisy breathing through failure to thrive. It may be present soon after birth with acute respiratory obstruction.

Congenital laryngeal stridor (laryngomalacia) is inspiratory and prominent during sleep. It is believed to be due to abnormally soft and floppy laryngeal structures. Stridor is worse on feeding and exertion.

Congenital
laryngeal
stridor

It is usually not a dangerous or significant condition, although worrying to parents. The condition disappeaars by the time that the child is 5 years old.

Laryngeal
paralysis

Laryngeal paralysis may result from birth trauma during difficult deliveries. It is caused by damage to the vagus nerve. It may lead to feeding difficulties. The condition tends to recover spontaneously in time.

Congenital
narrowing of
larynx

Congenital narrowing of the larynx may be caused by webs across the vocal cords or by subglottic cysts. These are difficult problems that require very skilled surgery which may be preceded by tracheostomy.

Croup (acute laryngitis)

Croup is a common specific syndrome in some children between 6 months and 3 years. There is a characteristic barking cough (like a dog or seal) that can be heard on the telephone or as soon as the doctor enters the house. The cough is worse at night between 11 pm and 2 am. The child is distressed with

crying, cough, fever and fright, but generally is bright. It causes
anxiety in the parents because of noise and the fear of suffoca-
tion. But once the doctor has visited and reassured, the child
almost always settles and sleeps after a warm drink. Next
morning there is little cough or stridor but the symptoms may
recur the next few nights.

Anxiety

Croup is caused by respiratory, syncytial and other viruses.
Antibiotics are not necessary. Dangerous features are a sickly,
quiet, whimpering child with severe breathing difficulties. He
must be admitted to hospital urgently.

Dangerous features

Acute epiglottitis

Acute epiglottitis is dangerous and potentially fatal. It is rare
but its possibility must be borne in mind. The epiglottis is
inflamed and oedema affects the epiglottis and the adjacent
supraglottic area.

The child is very ill with high fever and severe respiratory
distress. There is dysphagia with drooling of saliva from the
mouth, but cough and stridor are not prominent. The illness is
caused by *Haemophilus influenzae* type B.

Hospital admission

The child requires urgent hospital admission for relief of
airway obstruction and treatment by intravenous antibiotics
and steroids.

Note that acute epiglottitis can occur in adults with severe
sore throat, dysphagia and difficult breathing. The features and
pathology are similar to peritonsillitis (quinsy).

In adults

Multiple papillomata

Laryngeal papillomata (warts) occur in infants and children.
They are possibly caused by viruses. They can cause stridor
and persistent cough.

They disappear at puberty, but destruction by cryoprobe or
removal may be necessary.

Foreign bodies in trauma

Foreign bodies can cause stridor. A history of an inhaled
foreign body may be missing but the possibility must be borne
in mind.

79

Laryngeal diphtheria

This is now very rare but still is possible, particularly in non-immunized immigrant children.

Stridor

Stridor is produced by the flow of air through an *obstructed* upper airway.

Stridor most marked on inspiration is typical of an obstruction at the glottis or in the immediate sub-glottic region. Expiratory or biphasic stridor generally points to an obstruction below this level.

The obstruction causing stridor is potentially lethal as it may produce cardiorespiratory arrest from hypoxia and exhaustion.

The management of stridor is based on:

Diagnosis: – Infections account for 80% of stridor in children. 90% of this group are cases of laryngotracheobronchitis (croup) and 4% are epiglottitis. Inhalation of foreign body is another likely diagnosis of stridor of acute onset.

Accurate diagnosis is essential as the MANAGEMENT OF EACH CONDITION IS DIFFERENT. A foreign body requires endoscopic removal. The child with epiglottitis may suddenly become totally obstructed and an artificial airway ensures safety until antibiotics are effective. Laryngotracheobronchitis normally resolves with 'conservative' management and intubation is only required if the child becomes severely obstructed or exhausted.

A comparison between the presentation and signs of laryngotracheobronchitis and epiglottitis together with that for foreign body inhalation is shown in Table 12.1

Adults

Because of the larger size, laryngeal problems tend to cause hoarseness rather than stridor, certainly in the early stages of a disease. The two symptoms are parts of the same disorders.

Acute laryngitis

Acute laryngitis is usually part of a generalized upper respira-

Table 12.1 Two common forms of airway obstruction

	Subglottic infections (croup)	*Supraglottitis (epiglottitis)*
Incidence	Common 80% of stridor in children	Rarer 4% of stridor in children
Aetiological agent	Virus (parainfluenza, measles Rarely, *Haemophilus influenzae* or *Staphylococcus aureus*	*H. influenzae*–may be isolated from blood (50% or pharyngeal swab *S. aureus*
Age	6 months to 5 years; mmost <2 years old	Any age–can be seen in teenagers and adults–peak 2–6 years of age.
Onset	1–3 days; gradual; with upper respiratory tract infection	<24 hours; rapid
Symptoms	Croupy cough, symptoms of upper respiratory tract infection	Sore throat; inability to handle saliva; fever; lethargy; restlessness
Physical signs	Respiratory distress with inspiratory stridor	Upright position; head forward; tongue out; drooling; pallor; shock; restlessness; fever; respiratory distress; with retractions; high respiratory rate; muffled voice; inspiratory stridor; cyanosis, lethargy when severe
Leukocyte count	<10 k; lymphocytosis	>10 k; neutrophilia Band count high (>500)
Radiology	Anteroposterior and lateral neck on inspiration and expiration → narrowing of subglottic area	Lateral neck → swollen epiglottis (avoid manipulation of child)
Endoscopy	Subglottic inflammation, edema	Marked erythema, edema of epiglottis may be visible without laryngoscopy (avoid trauma)

Table 12.1   (Continued)

Treatment	Oxygen, fluids, humidity	Do nothing that makes it difficult for child to breathe
	intubation of severe obstruction ± steroids	Do not leave child alone
		Ventilate by mask when necessary
		Intubation (halothane.O_2) or tracheostomy–urgent
		Fluids, humidity, no sedatives before intubation
		Antibiotics ± steroids
Complications	Pulmonary edema Pneumonia Cardiac failure	Pneumonia Cervical lymphadenitis Tonsillitis Otitis media Pulmonary edema

Foreign body – There is a history of inhalation, coughing, choking, etc., typically in infants from 6 months of age to late childhood.
The clinical signs are croupy cough, respiratory distress, haemoptysis, wheezing (focal?) and hoarseness.
Investigations should be X-ray P/A and lateral chest, inspiratory and expiratory.

tory infection. The vocal cords have normal mobility but there is oedema and redness of the larynx. The condition often follows a common cold.

With symptomatic treatment (antibiotics not necessary) the condition should resolve within 2 weeks. If it persists then specialist referral is necessary.

'Chronic laryngitis'

'Chronic laryngitis' is not an infection but the result of misuse and abuse of the larynx by public speaking and singing (singer's nodes), smoking, alcohol drinking, the excessive eating of 'hot' foods (high temperature and curries, etc.). It is very rarely caused by true chronic infections such as tuberculosis or syphilis. The cords have normal mobility but they are thickened and white with red spots.

Nodules and polyps of the vocal cords are secondary to chronic laryngitis. The cords are mobile but there is oedema and redness with polypi or nodules.

Abuse and misuse of larynx

82

Management is by confirmation of diagnosis by a specialist, reassurance and advice on preventive measures.

Vocal cord paralysis

The immobile cord results from recurrent damage to laryngeal nerves. Lesions more often affect the left than the right nerve. Often no cause is found but possible causes are:

in chest

Causes in chest

cancers of bronchus and oesophagus,
mediastinal glands,
pulmonary tuberculosis,
aortic aneurysms,
chest surgery.

in neck

Causes in neck

thyroid cancer,
thyroid surgery,
malignant cervical glands,
cancer of hypopharynx.

Laryngeal neoplasms

These must be considered as a cause of hoarseness in an adult unless proved otherwise. If hoarseness persists longer than a month then referral to a specialist should be considered.

Benign tumours are rare and most laryngeal tumours are malignant. Malignant laryngeal tumours are classified by site in relation to the glottis, and can be:

Benign and malignant tumours

supraglottic,
glottic with the best prognosis,
subglottic,
pyriform fossa with hoarseness irlate.

Squamous cell carcinomata are most frequent in smoking males.

The larynx has abnormal mobility with an irregular mass and there is ulceration and oedema.

Treatment may include one or a combination of the following:–

Treatment

external irradiation,
surgery – total removal of larynx with or without block dissection of neck,
cytotoxic drugs.

Prognosis is good in 'early' cases, hence the importance of early diagnosis.

Chronic infections of larynx

Tuberculosis and syphilis is seen rarely.

Metabolic disorders

Some metabolic disorders affect the larynx such as hypothyroidism, and arthritis, especially when the cricoarytenoid joint is affected.

Trauma

Trauma to the vocal cords can result in haematoma and bruising. The mobility may be affected not only due to the oedema of the vocal cords but also its deformity.

Aphasia

Aphasia is a type of speech disorder where the patient has virtually no speech. It is caused by a lesion in the cortical speech centre or its connections.

The two common forms are auditory and visual aphasia

Auditory aphasia

In this condition there is loss of understanding of the spoken word although the hearing is normal.

Visual aphasia

With this disorder the patient cannot understand what is written, though possessing normal vision and normal spoken speech.

Aphonia

Aphonia (loss of voice) has either a functional (hysterical) or an organic cause.

Organic causes

The most common causes are due to disease of larynx. These may be inflammation, infection, trauma or neoplasm.

In addition to the nerve supply to the larynx may be damaged. This may be due either to a tumour of neck, trauma during thyroidectomy or stroke.

Dysarthria

This is a disturbance of speech and thus inability to articulate. Typically the consonants are affected more than vowels. It occurs when the function of lips, tongue or palate is affected independently or wholly.

Common causes

The most common causes are dental treatment, apthous ulcer, trauma to lips, tongue or palate, cleft palate.

There can also be CNS involvement, as in facial paralysis, poliomyelitis, tumours of base of brain, myasthenia gravis or Parkinson's disease.

13 Diplopia

Causes – Examination – Investigation

Diplopia is double vision. Occurs when two similar images are reproduced on two non-corresponding areas. One eye is unable to focus accurately on an object, which is clearly seen by the other.

Causes

Results from damage to or interference with functions of muscles and/or nerves controlling movements and focussing.

Common causes

The common causes are:

Trauma, i.e. facial fracture following road traffic accidents and sport injuries.

Orbital infection,

Frontal mucocoele – see Figure 13.1,

Tumour of nose and sinuses.

Oculomotor nerve involvement as in:
  (a) Raised intracranial pressure,
  (b) Brain stem lesion, e.g. disseminated sclerosis, tumours, vascular.

(c) Extracerebral lesion, e.g. aneurysm, meningitis, syndrome, nasopharyngeal carcinoma, trauma.

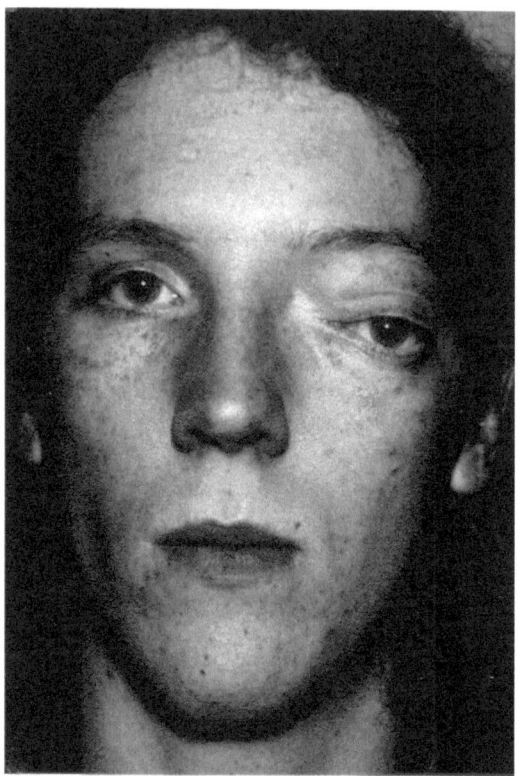

Diplopia due to a frontal mucocoele on the left side displacing the left orbit downwards and outwards

Figure 13.1

What to ask

History of trauma should be obtained.
Associated headaches and lethargy,
Pyrexia,
Severity of visual disturbances.

Examinations

Local   – Examination to determine the movements of the eye and involvement of adjacent structures.

General – A total examination should include central nervous system, cardiovascular system and exclude any metabolic disturbance.

Investigation

Blood films,
X-ray films.

In summary

Third cranial nerve damage
   Trauma – e.g. sports & road traffic accident injuries,
   Neoplasia,
   Multiple sclerosis,
   Causes of raised intracranial pressure,
   Infections, e.g. meningitis,
   Aneurysm.

Neuro muscular
   Myasthenia gravis,
   Thyrotoxicosis,
   Frontal osteoma or mucocoele,
   Neoplasia,
   Aneurysm.

14 Dysphagia

Causes – Types

Difficulty in swallowing may result from lesions along the length of the tract from the mouth to the stomach. (Figure 14.1).

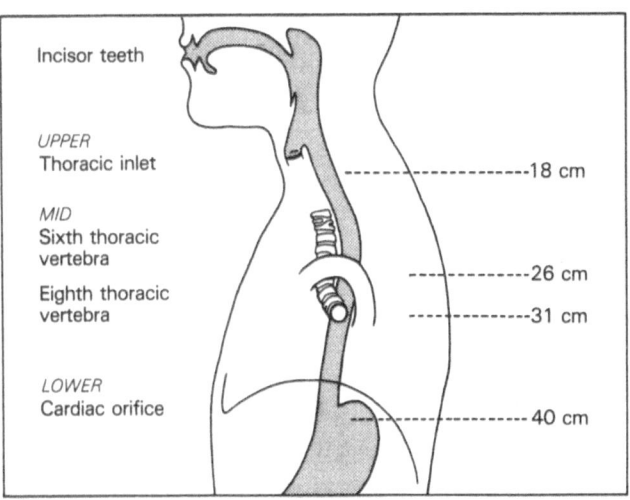

Diagram showing sites along oesophagus where lesions can occur and the length from the incisor teeth

Figure 14.1

The stages of swallowing are:

Chewing and passing the bolus to the back of the throat (upper level).

The swallowing reflex at the laryngo-pharyngeal (midlevel).

Involuntary progression through the oesophagus and entry into the stomach (lower levels).

Causes

Upper level

neuromuscular disorders,
neoplasms of tongue and pharynx,
pharyngeal pouch.

Mid-level

postcricoid carcinoma,
neuromuscular lesions (such as motor neuron disease, multiple sclerosis and cerebrovascular disease).

Lower level (oesophagus)

cancer,
benign strictures,
achalasia,
hiatus hernia and oesophagitis.

Types

Non-organic

'Globus hystericus' is a sensation of a constant lump in the throat, no loss of weight, no difficulties in swallowing and an anxious patient worrying over the possibility of cancer. It usually occurs in middle-aged women. The most effective management is to refer the patient to a specialist for reassurance.

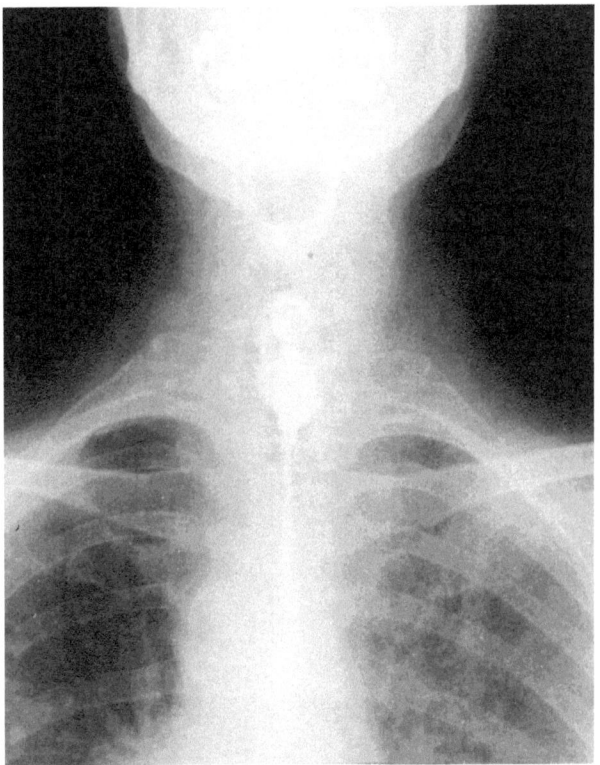

Strictures due to carcinoma of oesophagus – post-cricoid

Figure 14.2

Organic – serious

Postcricoid cancer (Figure 14.2) occurs in middle-aged women
with the syndrome of iron deficiency, koilonychia, glossitis
and angular stomatitis. This has many eponymous names:
Hurst–Plummer–Vinson and Paterson–Brown–Kelly syndromes.

Postcricoid
cancer

Before the appearance of the cancer there is a fibrous postcricoid web that itself causes dysphagia. The prognosis is poor
whatever the treatment.

Pyriform fossa cancer (Figure 14.3) is a condition of middle-
aged and elderly men. Dysphagia is a late symptom and does
not appear until the tumour is large enough to encroach on the
lumen of the food channel at this level.

Pyriform fossa
cancer

Earlier symptoms are hoarseness, earache and a lump in the
neck.

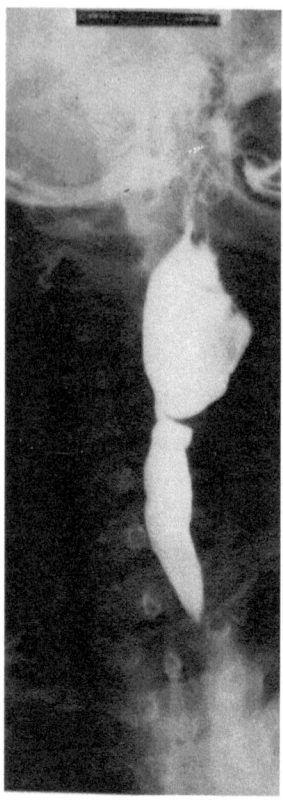

Figure 14.3

X-ray of a patient with pyriform fossa cancer

Treatment is with radiotherapy and cytotoxic drugs, or surgery involving radical laryngectomy and excision of the pharynx plus block dissection of the neck glands. The prognosis is poor.

Oesophageal cancer

Oesophageal cancer results in a narrowing of the oesophageal lumen and is fairly well localized. Early symptoms are of certain foods 'sticking' somewhere retrosternally, and later only slops or only fluids can be swallowed (Figure 14.4).

It is most prevalent in elderly men and again the prognosis is very poor.

Organic – not serious

Pharyngeal pouches occur in elderly men, particularly chronic

94

Pharyngeal
pouches

bronchitics. As the pouch enlarges food is regurgitated into the mouth. If untreated, enlargement may cause obstruction of the upper oesophagus and overspill lung infections (Figure 14.5).

Treatment is by endoscopic dilatation or surgical excision.

Benign
oesophageal
strictures

Benign oesophageal strictures develop from recurrent reflux oesophagitis, with or without hiatus hernia. With endoscopic dilatation and control off hyperacidity the outlook is very good.

Achalasia of
cardia

Achalasia of cardia is a neuromuscular dysfunction of the lower end of oesophagus and cardia. There is a pinch like appearance on X-ray. Dysphagia is at the lower part of the

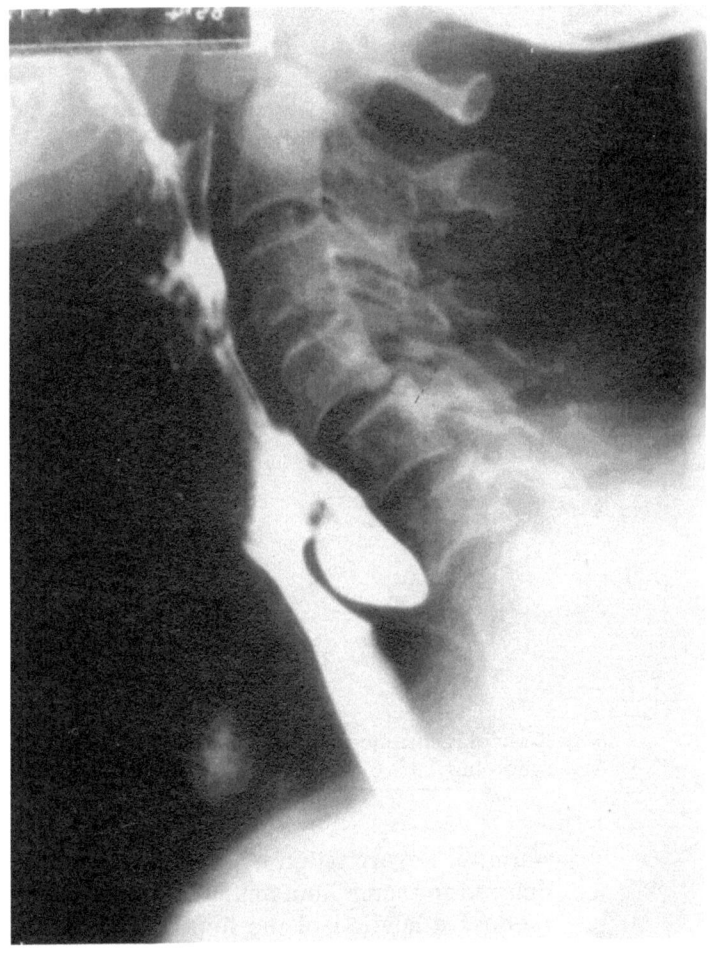

X-ray of a patient with pharyngeal pouch

Figure 14.4

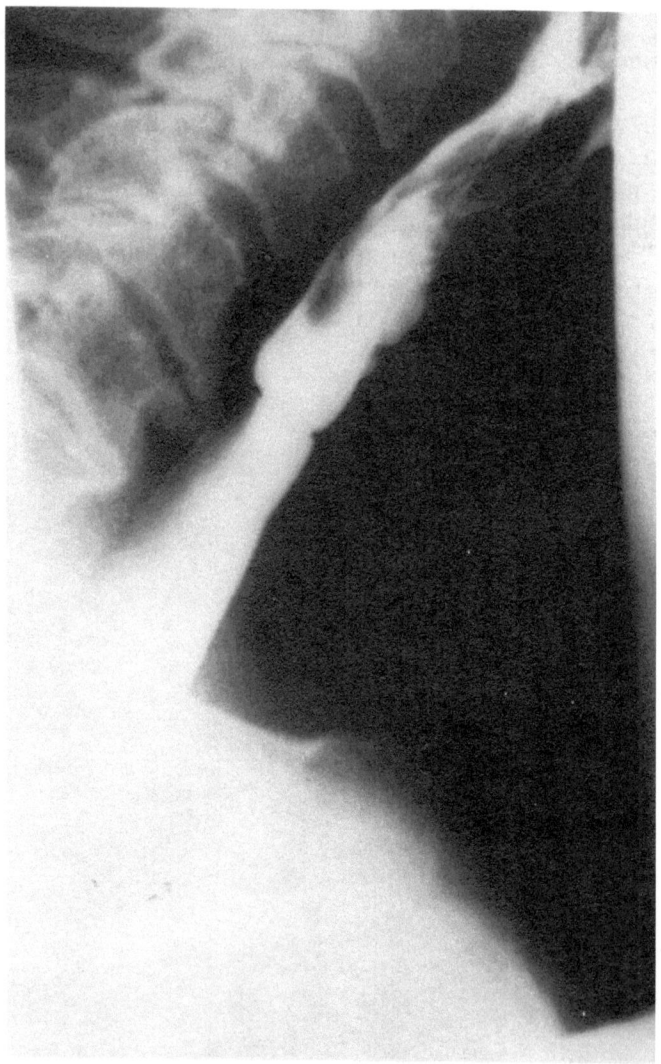

Figure 14.5

X-ray of recurrence of web in a patient with Patterson Brown-Kelly syndrome

sternum. Regurgitation of undigested food occurs but may be delayed for some hours after a meal.

Gross dilatation of the hypotonic oesophagus may lead to overspill resulting in lung infections.

Treatment with dilatation or cricopharyngeal myotomy produces good results, but recurrence may occur after dilatation.

15 Tonsils and adenoids

Who and when? – Why? – The catarrhal child syndrome – Effects – Tonsillectomy and/or adenoidectomy? – Indications – Results – Dangers

Removal of tonsils and adenoids is still carried out in one in five of all children and young adults. It is an operation shrouded in uncertainty and controversy. There are opponents and proponents. As always in medicine, there is no pure white or absolute black. The situation is a grey area requiring careful consideration of each case as to indications and likely benefits.

Who and when?

Tonsillectomy

The age distribution of tonsillectomy has a bipolar distribution. The operation is performed chiefly on children between 6 and 8 years, but there is a second peak in the teens and early twenties.

Adenoid ectomy

Adenoidectomy is entirely an operation of children between 3 and 8 years.

Why? (see also Indications)

The reasons generally given for the removal of tonsils and

97

adenoids are:

> repeated sore throats,
> recurrent 'sinusitis'
> enlarged cervical glands,
> persistent coughs and colds,
> recurrent otitis media,
> persistent deafness,
> many other reasons such as tuberculous adenitis, *Strep.* carriers, psoriasis, some autoimmune disorders.

The catarrhal child syndrome

The most prevalent disorder in children between 3 and 8 years comprises:

> recurrent coughs and colds,
> recurrent earache,
> recurrent sore throats,
> recurrent acute wheezy chests,
> persistent palpable cervical glands,
> persistent misery and malaise,
> anxious parents and grandparents,
> frustrated general practitioners,
> end-point ENT consultant faced with an opinion.

Symptoms

This syndrome has a characteristic natural history in that it resolves naturally after the age of 8, in the majority of cases, without any residual ill-effects.

Immunological reactions to environment

It is almost certain to be the effects of immunological reactions in growing children to noxious agents in the environment, such as, micro-organisms, atmosphere pollutants (particularly cigarette smoke) and climatic conditions.

Enlargement of glands

As a result of these situations the child's immature lymphatic reticuloendothelial system reacts. Since there is a large mass of lymphatic structures in the throat and neck, these are involved and react by inflammatory swelling – hence the enlargements of adenoids, tonsils and cervical glands.

Excessive secretion

Their swelling may cause obstruction of the Eustachian tube (adenoids) and other effects. As well as hypertrophy of lymphatic structures the respiratory tract responds by excessive secretion of mucus from nose, throat and bronchi (causing cough and wheezing).

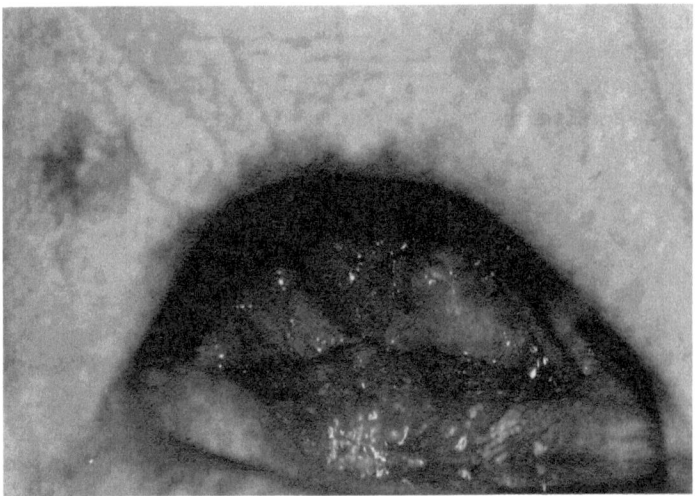

Carcinoma of lateral wall of pharynx extending into nasopharynx

Figure 15.1

Effects

Such changes produce clinical syndromes:

nasal discharge and obstruction ('colds'),
repeated swelling of tonsils ('tonsillitis'),
recurrent earache and deafness ('otitis media' and 'glue ear'),
palpable neck glands ('cervical adenitis'),
recurrent and persistent coughs with wheezing ('bronchitis' or 'asthma').

Why tonsillectomy and/or adenoidectomy?

(1) The rationale of removing tonsils and adenoids is that they are large, swollen and appear diseased.

(2) They are causing local complications such as otitis media and deafness from Eustachian tube dysfunction (blockage).

(3) They cause general ill health.

If such reasoning was followed completely then all children would have their tonsils and adenoids removed – as was almost the case among British middle and upper classes in the 1930's.

Indications

For the right reasons these surgical operations are some of the most gratifying. They do relieve symptoms, they do correct serious functional disabilities and they do improve general health.

Each child must be assessed individually but the following criteria should be used in making such assessments.

Adenoidectomy

(1) Persistent deafness following otitis media or without preceding acute attacks ('glue ear').

(2) Persistent and severe postnasal obstruction.

(3) As an accompaniment of tonsillectomy in children under 8.

Tonsillectomy

(1) Recurrent attacks of true tonsillitis, infection confined to tonsils (these are not common in young children).

(2) Recurrent attacks of true tonsillitis accompanied by general malaise, in young adults – particularly often infectious mononucleosis (glandular fever).

(3) Others must be rarely considered.

Results

The most satisfactory and dramatic results are observed in tonsillectomy in young adults and in adenoidectomy in deafness due to Eustachian tube dysfunction.

Dangers

Tonsillectomy and adenoidectomy, are not minor operations. Fortunately less than ten children die each year in Britain from these operations – but they are all normal children with normal abnormalities.

Probably in 5–10% of operations there are post-operative complications:

damage to teeth, uvula and palate,
laryngeal obstruction within an hour of the end of operation,
bleeding – reactionary (2–24 hours post-op), bleeding – secondary (7–10 days post-op).

16 Swellings of the neck

Congenital swellings – Inflammatory swellings – Neoplasm

Swellings of the neck can occur at any age group Figure 16.1 illustrates the rebative incidence of disease and size of lymph node to age. As much as the age may influence the diagnosis, management and subsequent prognosis, they all fall into one of the following groups:

Congenital	– e.g. cystic hygroma thyroglossal cyst
Inflammation	– e.g. cervical lymphadeno-pathy due to viral or bacterial infections
Infections	– e.g. Parapharyngeal abscess
Neoplasm Benign Malignant	carotid body lymphoma
Traumatic	– e.g. haematoma or emphysema following trauma to neck

The diagnosis and management of swellings of the neck is further enhanced by knowing the exact site of swelling when examining the patient. Figure 16.2 show the various triangles of the neck.

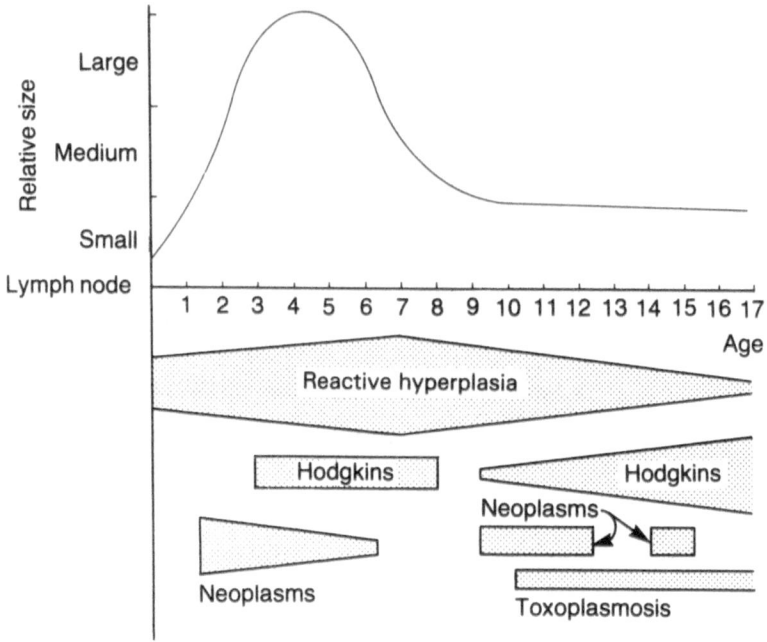

Graph to indicate size of lymph nodes to age and incidence of disease to age

Figure 16.1

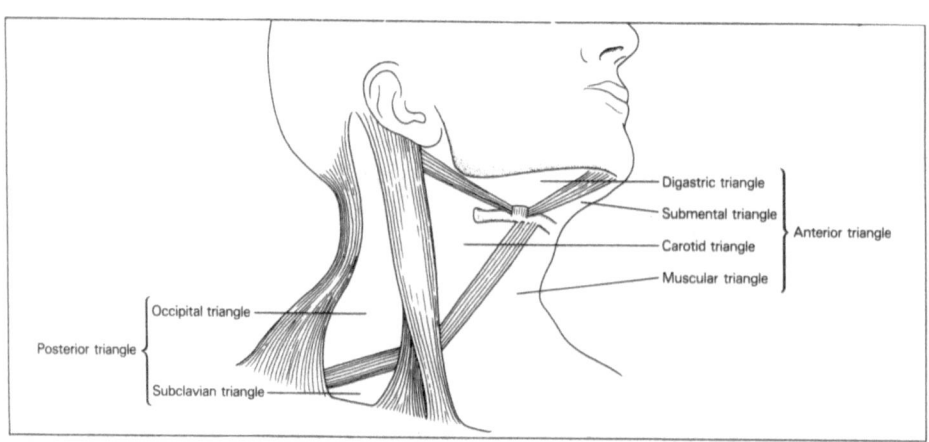

The triangles of the neck

Figure 16.2

Congenital swellings

Swellings may be either midline or lateral and are seen more often in the younger age group than the older.

The *midline swellings* present in the submental triangle or along the midline in relation to the hyoid cartilage, thyroid cartilage as far down the midline as the suprasternal notch, e.g.

Thyroglossal duct and cyst,
Dermoid,
Teratomas.

The *lateral neck swellings* present in the anterior triangle or posterior triangle are abnormalities of the branchial cleft, cystic hygroma, haemangiomas, and cysts of parotid, thyroid and thymus (Figure 16.3).

Branchial cleft abnormality may not manifest as a swelling till a much older age group and only when there is an infection. The infection is often the result of upper respiratory infection.

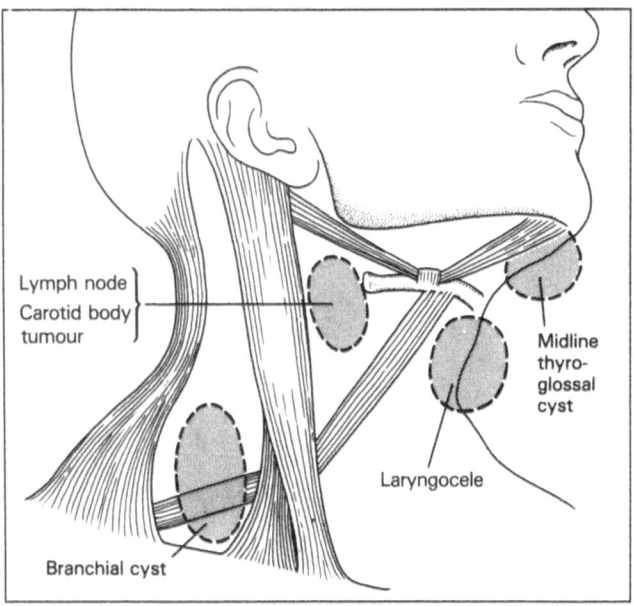

Sites of swellings in the neck

Figure 16.3 _____

Inflammatory swellings

Viral and bacterial infection are frequent causes of swellings in the neck. Enlargement of the cervical lymph nodes is most likely but a dormant branchial cyst may suddenly enlarge.

An understanding of the distribution of the superficial and deep cervical lymph nodes will help to arrive at a diagnosis (Figure 16.4).

Viral and bacterial infections that may cause cervical gland swellings are:

Infective mononucleosis,
Tonsillitis especially due to haemolytic strepococci,
Dental infections,
Para-pharyngeal infammatory process,
Tuberculosis,
Sarcoidosis.

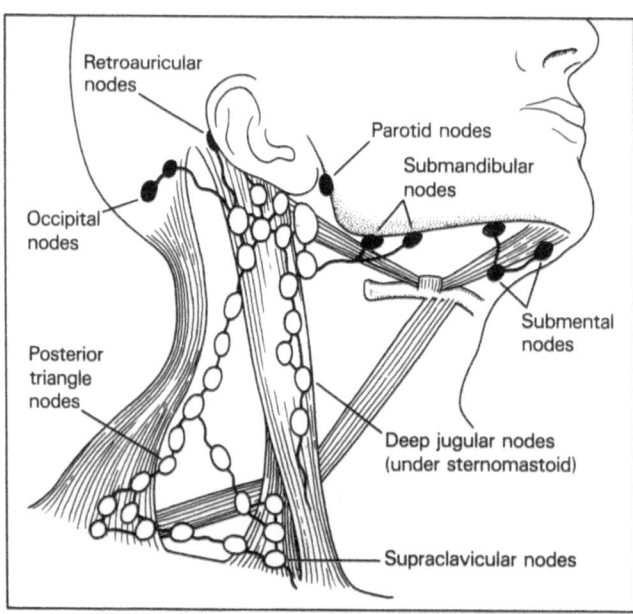

The main groups of lymph nodes of the neck

Figure 16.4

Neoplasm

Neoplasms that present as a swelling in the neck may be either benign or malignant.

Benign neoplasm arising in the neck as swellings are:

Haemangioma,
Lymphangioma,
Fibroma,
Lipoma,
Neurofibroma.

In the adult the same group of benign tumour are present but in addition there are chemodectomas, as the carotid body tumour.

The *carotid body tumour* presents a a non-tender mass at the bifurcation of the carotid artery increasing in size slowly. The characteristic feature of the lump is it can move in the horizontal plane, i.e. laterally but not in the vertical plane. The patient presents with cranial nerve lesions or dysphagia.

Malignant neoplasms in children are the lymphomas, sarcomas, and leukaemias. Carcinoma are of the thyroid gland, salivary gland and metastases from a primary growth in the head and neck, commonly the nasopharynx.

In the *adult* a swelling in the neck causes concern as it may be a metastasis. Hence the evaluation of a swelling in the neck in an adult must include a thorough clinical examination and investigation to exclude possible primary sites in lung, stomach, larynx, or mouth-pharynx.

What to do

If the history and clinical findings and investigations warrant treatment with antibiotics then immediate treatment should be commenced. If the practitioner has any doubts then the patient should be referred to the otolaryngologist or surgeon. An inflammatory or infective swelling resolves with treatment and hence there should be no delay in referring to the specialist if the swelling does not subside.

Index